SIRTFOOD DIET RECIPES

The Complete Guide to the New Revolutionary Weight Loss Diet. An Easy & Healthy Cookbook to Activate Your Skinny Gene, Burn Fat & Get Lean.

7-Days Meal Plan

Rebecca Right

Table of Contents

INTRODUCTION 3

CHAPTER 1: WHAT ARE SIRTFOODS?.. 6

CHAPTER 2: WHAT ARE SIRTUINS? 9

CHAPTER 3: HOW DO SIRTFOOD DIETS WORK? 15

CHAPTER 4: WHO IS IT FOR? 18

CHAPTER 5: LIST OF SIRTFOODS 20

CHAPTER 6: HOW MANY SIRTFOODS DO YOU NEED TO EAT? 30

CHAPTER 7: SIRTUIN DIET PLAN 34

CHAPTER 8: BREAKFASTS RECIPES.. 41

CHAPTER 9: JUICES AND SMOOTHIES.. 73

CHAPTER 10: PHASE 1 RECIPES.. 91

CHAPTER 11: PHASE 2 RECIPES... 113

CHAPTER 12: 7-DAYS MEAL PLAN.. 123

CHAPTER 13: DESSERTS RECIPES 127

CHAPTER 14: BONUS RECIPE 151

CONCLUSION 174

Introduction

There's no denying that sirtfoods benefit you. They are frequently high in nutrients and complete healthy plant compounds. Moreover, research studies have associated many of the foods recommended on the Sirtfood Diet with health advantages.

For example, consuming moderate amounts of dark chocolate with high cocoa content might decrease the danger of cardiovascular disease and assistance fight inflammation. Consuming green tea might decrease the risk of stroke and diabetes and help lower high blood pressure, and turmeric has anti-inflammatory properties that have beneficial impacts on the body in general and may even secure against chronic, inflammation-related illness).

For instance, researchers have found that increased levels of specific sirtuin proteins cause a longer lifespan in yeast, mice, and worms. And throughout fasting or calorie limitation, sirtuin proteins inform the body to burn more fat for energy and improve insulin level of sensitivity. One study in mice discovered that increased sirtuin levels resulted in weight loss.

Some evidence recommends that sirtuins may likewise play a role in minimizing swelling, hindering the advancement of growths, and slowing the development of cardiovascular disease and Alzheimer's.

While research studies in mice and human cell lines have revealed favorable results, no human studies are examining the increasing sirtuin levels. Whether increasing sirtuin protein levels in the body will lead to a longer lifespan or a lower danger of cancer in humans is unknown.

A research study is currently underway to develop substances efficient at increasing sirtuin levels in the body. By doing this, human research studies can begin to take a look at the effects of sirtuins on human health

Until then, it's not possible to identify the results of increased sirtuin levels.

Sirtfoods are generally healthy foods. Extremely little is understood about how these sirtfoods affect sirtuin levels and human health. Sirtfoods are nearly all healthy options and may even lead to some health benefits due to their anti-inflammatory or antioxidant residential or commercial properties.

Yet consuming only healthy foods can not satisfy all of your body's dietary needs. The Sirtfood Diet is needlessly restrictive and uses no clear and unique health benefits over any other kind of diet.

Eating only 1,000 calories usually is not suggested without the supervision of a physician. Even consuming 1,500 calories per day is exceedingly limiting for many individuals.

What's more, sipping on juice throughout the whole day is a wrong concept for both your blood sugar and your teeth. Not to point out, because the diet plan is so minimal in calories and food choice, it is more than most likely lacking in protein, vitamins, and minerals, specifically during the first stage.

This diet plan may be challenging to adhere to for the whole three weeks. Add to this the high initial expenses of needing to buy a juicer, book, and specific uncommon and costly components, and the time expenses of making specific meals and juices. This diet plan ends up being unrealistic and unmanageable for many individuals.

The Sirtfood Diet promotes healthy foods but is limiting in calories and food choices. It likewise involves drinking great deals of juice, which isn't a healthy suggestion.

Yet for somebody with diabetes, calorie limitation and drinking primarily juice for the very first couple of days of the diet might cause hazardous modifications in blood glucose levels. Even a healthy individual may experience some side results—generally hunger.

Eating just 1,000–1,500 calories per day will leave practically anybody sensation starving, mainly if much of what you're taking in is juice, which is low in fiber. This nutrient helps keep you feeling complete. Throughout phase one, you might experience opposite effects such as fatigue, irritability, and lightheadedness due to the calorie limitation.

For the otherwise healthy adult, significant health consequences are unlikely if the diet plan is followed for just three weeks. The Sirtfood Diet is low in calories and phase one is not nutritionally well balanced. It may leave you hungry; however, it's not harmful to the average healthy grownup.

Chapter 1: What Are Sirtfoods?

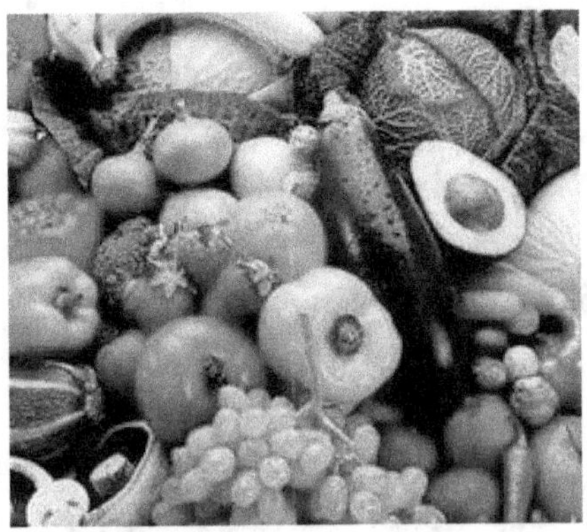

Sirtfoods are a particular type of food that is high in sirtuin activators. They contain a type of protein that helps to protect the cells in the body and prevent the cells from dying or becoming inflamed through illnesses. The protein present in sirtfood also helps to regulate the body metabolism, increase muscles as well as burning of fat.

Sirtfood foods are rich in sirtuins. They contain a specialized type of protein and they help to burn fat, regulate metabolism and increase muscle weight.

The Sirtfood diet primarily emphasizes the consumption of foods that contain a group of proteins known as sirtuin. Thus, the name Sirtdiet is authored from the sirtuin protein. Sirtfood eats less carbs are likewise known for their extraordinary capacity to ensure against malignant growth, improve memory, and control glucose levels. The first Sirtfood Diet book was published in 2016 in the United Kingdom. The sirtfood diet began to gain popularity when a world-known celebrity "Adele" showcased her slimmer figure at the Billboard Music Competition. She made it known that her trainer, Pete Geracimo, is a fan of the sirtfood diet and how the singer lost about 30 pounds from using the sirtfood diet. Sirtfood is very useful for burning fat, weight loss, healthy lifestyle and boosting your muscles, and energy level.

How Does Sirtfood Work?

Getting fit and losing weight could be very simple and straightforward if only you do the right thing. One way is to create a meal timetable that calorie deficit either by increasing your burning of calorie through workouts or reducing your intake of calories

In the year 2015, a pilot study was carried out by Goggin's and Matten. They tested the effectiveness of sirtuins using people for the sample studies. The people that participated in the experiment lost about seven pounds in just seven days. Those results were awe-inspiring. However, some Weight-loss experts also have some doubts about the lofty promises. However, these claims are highly speculative and extrapolate from studies carried out in simple organisms such as yeast at the cellular levels. It is important to note that whatever happens at the cellular level does not necessarily translate to what happens in the human body at the macro level.

What Does the Diet Entail?

The diet is used in two phases. The first phase can last for three days and also restricts calories to about 1,000 per day. Usually, it consists of three green juices and one sirtfood approved meal. While the second phase can last for four days and can raise the daily allotment to about 1,500 calories per day with about two green juices and two meals

After these phases have been achieved, there is a need to carry out a maintenance plan. This maintenance plan isn't focused on calories instead it is based on sensible portions, well-balanced diets, and engaging primarily sirtfoods. You will be required to carry out a 14 days maintenance plan featuring three meals: one with green juice and one or two with sirtfood bite snacks.

Benefit of Sirtfood

- **Weight loss:** You will lose a lot of weight if you follow this diet strictly. It does not matter whether you are eating 1,000 calories of tacos or 1,000 calories of kale or 1,000 calories of snicker doodles. What you should know is that you will lose weight at 1,000 calories. However, you will be more successful when you carry out some amount of calorie restriction. If your daily caloric intake is between 2,000 to 2,200, you may need to reduce it to 1,500 for an effective weight-loss strategy.

Precautions to Be Taken

This plan may be a bit strict with little wiggle room or substitutions. Weight loss can be maintained if a low caloric intake is maintained, this may make it challenging to adhere to long-term. This simply means that any weight lost in the first seven days is most likely to be gained back at the end of the exercise.

Chapter 2: What Are Sirtuins?

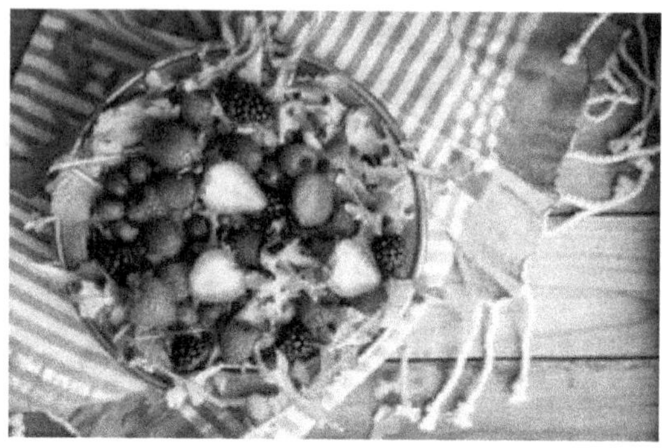

Sirtuins are among the family of proteins that function to regulate cellular health, including homeostasis. Hemostasis is the process by which the body maintains stability, adjusts the conditions that are best for survival. The SIRT protein family has seven members (SIRT1-7). SIR2 yeast silent information regulator is the founding member of the SIRT protein family that controls chromatin, DNA recombination, and gene expression. Among the seven mammalian SIRTs, SIRT1, SIRT2, and SIRT3 have the ability to deacetylase.

Other remaining SIRTs (SIRT4, SIRT5, SIRT6, and SIRT7) possess a weak or no detectable deacetylates activity. SIRT1-7 differs in function and cellular localization. SIRT1 is located in the cytosol and nucleus where it performs its function for cellular life. It is involved in glucose metabolism, neurodegeneration, and differentiation, control of Gene expression, aging, cell death, and tumorigenesis. SIRT2, located in the cytosol, helps to catalyze the deacetylation of Alpha tubulin (Lys40), H31ys56, FOXO1, H41ys16, and FOXO3a.

In addition to that, it is involved in Gene expression regulation, tubulin acetylation, tubulin acetylation, cell cycle regulation, DNA damage response, cancer, neurodegeneration. SIRT3 location in mitochondria inner membrane with substrates of long-chain acyl-CoA dehydrogenase

(LCDA), acetyl-CoA synthetase 2 (ACS2), 2, 3-hydroxy-3-methylglutaryl CoA synthetase 2 (HMGCS2), ornithine trans carbamoyltransferase (OTC), glutamate dehydrogenase (GDH), Cycle-Philip D, superoxide dismutase 2(SOD2), isocitrate dehydrogenase 2 (IDH2), numerous components of the mitochondria respiratory chain complexes as well as Ku70. It is responsible for mitochondria ATP production, fatty acid oxidation, as well as regulation of mitochondrial protein.

Also, it controls caloric restriction and cellular response to oxidative stress through the activation of SOD2 and IDH2, which will reduce oxidized reactive oxygen species (ROS) and glutathione. It also involved in tumor suppression and cell death, thereby influencing genomic stability positively. SIRT4 is located in the Mitochondrial Matrix. It is involved in ADP-ribosylation and GHD inhibition by utilizing NAD+. SIRT5, also localized in the mitochondrial Matrix, contains an NAD+ dependent decarboxylase as well as desuccinylase activity on CPS1. SIRT6, functioning as deacetylase, and ADP-ribosyl transferase is necessary for telomeric functions, metabolism hemostasis, DNA repair, and genome stability. SIRT7 is a predominantly nucleolar protein that regulates the transcription of the ribosomal genes by interacting with RNA polymerase 1. SIRT7 has high selectivity for the H31ys18 and also has a NAD+ dependent deacetylase. When SIRT7 gets deacetylated, we need to repression of genes that are involved in cellular Anchorage and contact inhibition, thereby favoring the malignant phenotype tumor cells.

The Sirtfood Science

The sirtfood diet can't be classified as low-carb or low-fat. This diet is quite different from its many precursors while advocating many of the same things: the ingestion of fresh plant-based foods. As the name implies, this is a sirtuin-based diet, but what are sirtuins, and why have you never heard about them before?

There are seven sirtuin proteins—SIRT-1 to SIRT-71. They can be found throughout your cells and the cells of every animal on the planet. Sirtuins are found in almost every living organism and almost every part of the cell, controlling what goes on. Supplement company Elysium Health, likens the body's cells to an office with sirtuins acting as the CEO, helping the cells react to internal and external changes. They govern what is done, when it's done, and who does it.

Of the seven sirtuins, one works in your cell's cytoplasm, three in the cell's mitochondria, and another three in the cell's nucleus. They have a full number of jobs to perform, but mostly they remove acetyl groups from other proteins. These acetyls groups signal that the protein they are attached to is available to perform its function. Sirtuins remove the available flag and get the protein ready to use.

Sirtuins sound pretty crucial to your body's normal function, so why have you never heard of them before?

The first sirtuin to be discovered was SIR2, a gene discovered in the 1970s which controlled the ability of fruit flies to mate. It wasn't until the 1990s that scientists discovered other, similar proteins, in almost every form of life. Every organism had a different number of sirtuins—bacteria has one and yeast has five. Experiments on mice show they have the same number than humans, seven.

Sirtuins have been shown to prolong life in yeast and mice. There is no evidence of the same effect in human beings; however, these sirtuins are present in almost every form of life and many scientists are hopeful that if organisms as far apart as yeast and mice can see the same effect from sirtuin activation, this may also extend to humans.

In addition to sirtuins, our bodies need another substance called nicotinamide adenine dinucleotide for cells to function correctly. Elysium (see above) likens this substance to the money a company needs to keep operating. Like any CEO, a sirtuin can only keep the company working correctly if the cash flow is sufficient. NAD+ was first discovered in 1906. You get your supply of NAD+ from your diet by eating foods made up the building blocks of NAD+.

Fun Facts about Sirtuins

1. Mice that have been engineered to have high levels of SIRT-1 are both more active and leaner than average, while mice that lack SIRT-1 altogether are fatter and more prone to various metabolic conditions.

2. Add the fact that levels of SIRT-1 are much lower in obese people than in those of a "healthy" weight, and the case for the importance of sirtuins in weight loss becomes compelling.

3. By changing your diet and adding the best sirtfoods to your eating plan; the authors of the sirtfood diet believe everyone can achieve better health without losing muscle mass.

The Sirtfood for Weight Loss

Research conducted by Aidan Goggin's and Glen Martin showed that 7 pounds of weight were lost on average in seven days on the Sirt food diet after taking note of muscle gain. Sirtuins' diet has not promised only weight loss; instead, good health as well. An increase in the level of body sirtuins has been proven to cause weight loss. The best way of increasing body leptin is still through fasting and exercise. Also, one of the best ways of enhancing body sirtuins is by consumption of sirtuin foods. All the seas will affect the body's metabolism.

Furthermore, hypothalamic SIRT1 has been proven to help in weight loss. The hypothalamus is the central weight and energy balance controller. It modulates energy intake and energy consumption by neural inputs from the periphery, as well as direct humor inputs, which sense the energy status of the body. An adipokine, leptin, is one of the factors that signal that sufficient energy is stored on the periphery. Leptin plasma levels are favorable for adiposity, suppressing energy intake, and stimulating energy spending.

A prolonged increase in the level of plasma leptin in obese can cause leptin resistance. Leptin resistance can affect the hypothalamus from having access to leptin, which also reduces leptin signal transduction in the hypothalamic neurons. Reduced peripheral energy-sensing by leptin can lead to a positive energy balance and incremental weight gain and adiposity improvements, which further exacerbate leptin resistance.

Leptin resistance causes an increase in adiposity, just like weight gain, all of which are associated with aging. Similar observations occur in central insulin resistance. The improvement of the action of humoral factors in the hypothalamus can, therefore, prevent progressive weight gains, especially among middle-aged individuals. SIRT1 is a protein deacetylase, NAD+ dependent, which has many substrates, such as transcription factors, histones, co-factors, and various enzymes. SIRT1 improves the sensitivity to leptin and insulin by decreasing the levels of several molecules that impair the transduction of leptin and insulin signals.

The hypothalamic SIRT1 and NAD+ levels decrease with age. It has been shown that an increase in the level of SIRT1 improves the level of conservation in mice and so prevents age-related weight gain. By preventing the loss of age-dependent SIRT1 hypothalamus role, there will be a boost in the activity of humoral factors in the hypothalamus and the central energy balance control.

Sirtfood for Building Muscle

Sirtuins are a group of proteins with different effects. Sirt-1 is the protein responsible for causing the body to burn fat rather than muscle for energy, which is a miracle for weight loss. Another useful aspect of Sirt-1 is its ability to improve skeletal muscle.

Skeletal muscle is all the muscles you voluntarily control, such as the muscles in your limbs, back, shoulders, and so on. There are two other types, cardiac muscle is what the heart is formed of, while a smooth muscle is your involuntary muscles—which includes muscles around your blood vessels, face and various parts of organs, and other tissues.

Skeletal muscle is separated into two different groups, the blandly named type-1 and type-2. Type 1 muscle is active at continued, sustained activity whereas type-2 muscle is active at short, intense periods of activity. So, for example, you would predominantly use type-1 muscles for jogging, but type-2 muscles for sprinting.

Sirt-1 protects the type-1 muscles, but not the type-2 muscle, which is still broken down for energy. Therefore, holistic muscle mass drops when fasting, even though type-1 skeletal muscle mass increases.

Sirt-1 also influences how the muscles work. Sirt-1 is produced by the muscle cells, but the ability to produce Sirt-1 decreases as the muscle ages. As a result, muscle is harder to build as your age and doesn't grow as fast in response to exercise. A lack of sirt-1 also causes the muscles to become tired quicker and gradually decline over time.

When you consider these effects of sirt-1, you can form a picture about why fasting helps keep the body supple. Fasting releases sirt-1, which helps skeletal muscle grow and stay in good shape. Sirt-1 is also released by consuming sirtuin activators, giving the sirtfood diet its muscle retaining power.

Chapter 3: How Do Sirtfood Diets Work?

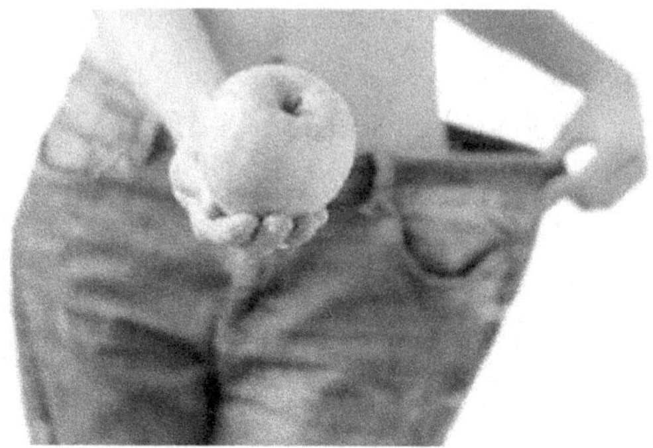

We've learned so far that sirtuins are an ancient gene family with the ability to help us burn fat, build muscle, and keep us super happy. It is well known that by caloric restriction, fasting, and exercise, sirtuins can be turned on. Still, there is another innovative way to achieve this: diet. We refer to the most active foods to activate sirtuins as Sirtfoods.

To understand the benefits of Sirtfoods, we need to learn about foods like fruits and vegetables very differently, and why they are perfect for us. Despite tons of evidence demonstrating that diets high in fruits, vegetables, and plant foods usually cut the risk of many chronic diseases, including the biggest killers, heart disease, and cancer, there is absolutely no doubt they do. This has been put down to their rich nutrient content, such as vitamins, minerals, and, of course, antioxidants, which is probably the greatest wellness buzzword of the last decade. But this is a very different story we are here to share.

The explanation why Sirtfoods is so fantastic for you has nothing to do with the nutrients we all know so well and hear about so much about. Yes, they're all valuable things you need to get out of your diet. Still, with Sirtfoods there's something entirely different and very unique. In reality, what if we turned that whole way of thinking on its ear and said that the explanation the Sirtfoods is right for you is not because they nourish the body or because they provide antioxidants to mop up the damaging effects of free radicals, but quite the opposite: because they are full of weak toxins? This might sound crazy in an environment where almost every alleged "healthy food" is aggressively marketed focused on its antioxidant content. But it's a revolutionary idea and one worth taking on.

What Makes You Stronger

Let's get back for a moment to the proven methods of triggering sirtuins: fasting and exercise. Evidence has shown consistently, as we have seen, that the allocation of dietary resources has significant effects on weight loss, wellbeing, and, quite likely, lifespan. Then there is fitness, with its numerous advantages for both body and mind, pointed out by the discovery that regular exercise slashes mortality rates dramatically. But what is the one thing they have in common?

The answer lies in heat. All fasting and exercise cause the body to experience moderate stress that helps it to adjust by becoming more robust, more productive, and more durable. It is the reaction of the body to these slightly unpleasant stimuli—its adaptation—that, in the long run, should make us better, safer, and leaner. So, as we now learn, sirtuins orchestrate these highly beneficial modifications, which are turned on in the presence of these stressors, so spark a series of desirable changes in the body.

The technical term used to respond to those pressures is hormesis. It's the theory that if subjected to a low dose of a drug or stimulus that is otherwise harmful or fatal if administered at higher doses, you get a beneficial effect. Perhaps "things that don't kill you make you stronger," and that's how fasting works because hunger is fatal, so excessive exercise is prejudicial to safety. Such extreme forms of stress are inherently dangerous. Still, they have highly beneficial consequences, as well as diet and activity, to stay mild and controlled pressures.

Enter Polyphenols

So, here's where things get interesting. Many living organisms undergo hormesis, but the reality that this also involves plants is what has been highly undervalued until now. Although we would not typically think of plants as being the same as other living organisms, let alone humans, we do share similar responses in terms of how we respond to our environment on a chemical level.

As mind-blowing as that is, it makes perfect sense to think evolutionary about it because all living things have adapted to encounter and deal with specific environmental pressures such as starvation, heat, lack of nutrition, and pathogens assault.

If it is hard for you to wrap your head around, get ready for that truly amazing part. Reactions to plant tension are, in general, more complex than ours. Think about it: if we're hungry and thirsty, we can go in search of food and drink; it's too humid, we're in the shade; we can escape under assault. By complete contrast, plants are stagnant, and all the effects of these physiological pressures and challenges will survive. Their influence is profound: they activate our inherent receptors to react to stress. Here we are talking about precisely the same directions that turn on to fasting and exercise: the sirtuins. Piggybacking on the stress-response system of a plant in this fashion is regarded as xenohormesis for our gain.

The implications of that are game-changing. Nevertheless, because of their ability to turn on the same positive changes in our bodies, such as fat burning, that would be visible during fasting, these natural plant compounds are now referred to as reflective caloric constraints, and by supplying us with more sophisticated signaling compounds than we are generating ourselves, they cause effects comparable to anything that can be obtained by eating or exercising alone.

Chapter 4: Who Is It for?

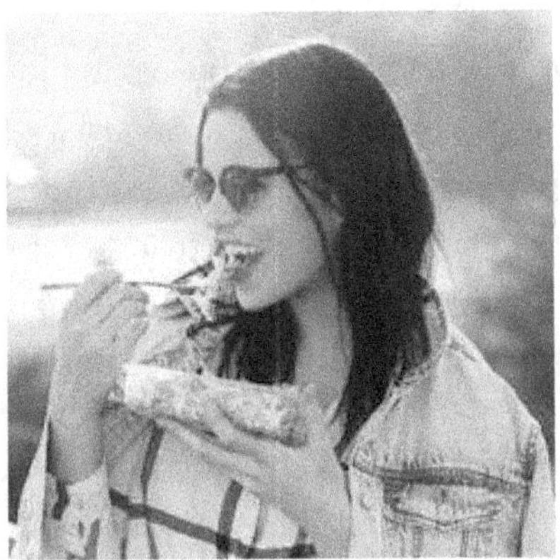

Anyone who can make the best use out of this diet should try it. There is no one formula of who should try the sirtfood diet and who shouldn't. However, based on the body's needs and the physical problems a person is suffering from, we can decide on a better utility of this diet. Following are the cases in which the sirtfood diet can prove to be most effective.

1. **Obesity:** Sirtuin burns fats quickly, and that's what makes this diet an excellent help for weight loss. When we study all the cases of successful sirtfood dieters, we can see how well they fought against obesity. Adele is just one example, who has amazed the world with her 30 pounds of weight loss achievement using the sirtfood diet. So, anyone who isn't able to lose some extra pounds for whatever reason, can switch to sirtfood and then can see the magic happening.

2. **Low or poor metabolic activity:** Since sirtuins are mainly responsible for better cell metabolism, lower sirtuin levels in the body can hamper natural cell activities and hinders metabolism. Reduced metabolic activity results in weakening of physical strength, obesity, hormonal imbalance, low enzymic activity, and several other related problems. The sirtfood diet is therefore

suggested to boost the metabolic rates in the body and revitalize the body and the mind with levels of energy.

3. **No workouts:** Extraneous workouts are just not for everybody. Sure, working out is an excellent way to lose some pounds. Still, every other person can't invest the required time and energy into the workouts. Therefore, the sirtfood diet can be used by such individuals. Through this diet, they can manage their weight and lose it even while doing some necessary physical activities.

4. **Aging:** Aging seems like a threat to all when those wrinkles start appearing on the skin, and the person feels weakened inside out! Well, this magic gene sirtuin can also play its part in countering the effects of aging. It helps DNA to prolong its life and also aid in the repair process. Sirtuin is also responsible for apoptosis and leads to the formation of new healthy cells. This is the reason why people who are entering middle age should consider doing the sirtfood diet so that they could effectively fight the possible signs of aging in the coming years.

5. **Inflammation:** What appears to be weight gain or metabolic inactivity is mostly connected to inflammation of both cells and organs in most cases. This inflammation is both the result and cause of several health problems. Sirtfood does not only prevent inflammation at cellular levels, but effectively prevents it at the tissue and organ level.

6. **Stress:** There is one added advantage that higher sirtuin levels can guarantee and that is the reduction in stress and depression. Research is still being conducted on the relationship between sirtfood and stress. Still, sirtuin is that element that can enable quick brain cell recovery and boosts brain activity by getting rid of all the unwanted metabolic waste. Efficient brain functioning then leads to a reduction in stress. So, this sirtfood diet can also help with stress relief.

Chapter 5: List of Sirtfoods

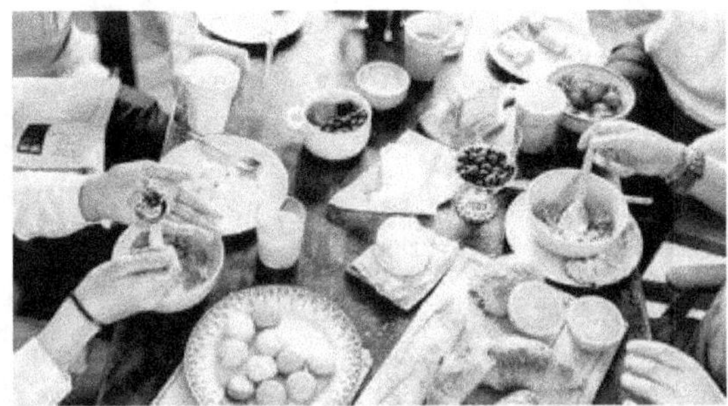

- **Arugula:** arugula (also known as a missile, rucola, rugula, and roquette) has a vivid background of American culinary culture. A pungent green salad leaf with a distinctive peppery flavor soon ascended from humble beginnings as the base of many Mediterranean peasant dishes to becoming an emblem of food snobbery in the United States, thus contributing to the coining of the word arugulance!

- **Buckwheat:** Buckwheat was one of Japan's first domesticated grains, and the legend goes that when Buddhist monks took long journeys into the mountains, they'd only bring a cooking pot and a buckwheat bag for warmth. Buckwheat is so good that this was all they wanted, and it kept them up for weeks. We're huge fans of buckwheat too. Firstly, since it is one of a sirtuin activator's best-known origins, named rutin. But also, because it has benefits as a cover crop, enhancing soil fertility and reducing weed growth, making it a perfect crop for environmentally friendly and sustainable agriculture.

- **Capers:** In case you're not so familiar with capers, we're talking about the spicy, dark green, pellet-like stuff on top of a pizza that you may never have had occasion to see. But yes, they are one of the most undervalued and neglected foods out there. Intriguingly, they are the caper bush's flower buds that grow abundantly in the Mediterranean before being picked and preserved by hand. Studies now show that capers possess essential antimicrobial, antidiabetic, anti-inflammatory, immunomodulatory, and antiviral properties, and have a long tradition of being used as a medicine in the Mediterranean and North Africa. It's hardly shocking when we find they are filled with nutrients that trigger sirtuin.

- **Celery:** For millennia, Celery has been present and revered—leaves have been found adorning the remains of the Egyptian pharaoh Tutankhamun, who died around 1323 BCE. Early varieties were very bitter, and Celery was commonly considered a medicinal plant, particularly for washing and detoxification to prevent disease. This is especially interesting considering that protecting the liver, kidneys, and intestines is one of the many positive benefits.

- **Chilies:** Chili has been an essential part of gastronomic history worldwide for thousands of years. At one point, it's disconcerting that we'd be so enamored by it. Its pungent fire, caused by a substance called capsaicin in chilies, is developed as a mechanism of plant defense to inflict pain and dissuade predators from feasting on it, and we appreciate that. The food and our infatuation with it are almost magical.

- **Cocoa:** Cocoa has fantastic health benefits. It's no surprise to hear that cocoa was considered a holy food for ancient cultures like the Aztecs and Mayans, and was typically reserved for the powerful and the soldiers consumed at feasts to win allegiance and service. Indeed, there was such high respect for the cocoa bean that it was also used as a form of currency. It was typically served as a frothy beverage back then. Yet what might be a tastier way to get our dietary allowance of cacao than by chocolate? Unfortunately, there's no count here for the condensed, aged, and chemically sweetened milk chocolate we usually munch. We're talking of chocolate with 85 percent solids of cocoa to earn the Sirtfood tag.

- **Coffee:** What's all that about Sirtfood Coffee? We know whatever you're thinking. We will tell you that there is no mistake. Gone are the days when a twinge of remorse had to balance our enjoyment of coffee. Evidence is unambiguous: coffee is a healthy food that is bona fide. Indeed, it is a real treasure chest of fantastic nutrients that trigger sirtuin. And with more than half of Americans consuming coffee every day (to the tune of $40 billion a year!), coffee enjoys the accolade of becoming America's number one source of polyphenols. The biggest irony is that the only thing we were chastised by so many fitness "experts" for doing was, in essence, the best thing we were doing about our wellbeing each day.

- **Extra-virgin olive oil:** Olive oil is the most popular of Mediterranean traditional diets. The olive tree is among the world's oldest-known planted plants, also known as the "immortal tree." And after people began pressing olives in stone mortars to harvest them, the oil has been worshipped, almost 7,000 years ago. Hippocrates cited it as a cure-all; today, a few decades' future use, scientific medicine confidently claims the beautiful health effects. There is now a wealth of scientific data showing that regular olive oil consumption is powerfully cardioprotective.

- **Garlic:** Garlic has been considered one of nature's miracle foods for thousands of years, with soothing and rejuvenating properties. Egyptians feed pyramid workers with garlic to enhance their immunity, avoid various illnesses, and strengthen their performance by resisting fatigue. Garlic is a potent natural antibiotic and antifungal that is sometimes used to help cure ulcers in the stomach. Promoting the elimination of waste materials from the body will activate the lymphatic system to "detox." Besides being researched for weight reduction, it also delivers a potent heart safety punch, reducing cholesterol by around 10 percent, lowering blood pressure by 5 to 7 percent, and lowering blood and blood sugar stickiness.

- **Green tea (Matcha in particular):** Many would be familiar with green tea, the toast of the Orient and ever more common in the West. With the increasing awareness of its health benefits, green tea intake is related to less cancer, heart disease, diabetes, and osteoporosis. It is believed that green tea is so healthy for us that it is primarily due to its rich content of a group of healthy plant compounds called catechins, the star of the show being a unique form of sirtuin-activating catechin known as epigallocatechin gallate (EGCG).

- **Kale:** We are at heart cynics, so we are always skeptical about what drives the latest craze for superfood advertising. Is it science, or are its interests at stake? In recent years, few foods have exploded as dramatically as kale on the health scene. Described as the "lean, green brassica queen" (referring to its cruciferous vegetable family), it has become the chic vegetable for which all health-lovers and foodies are gunning. Each October, there is also a National Day of the Kale. But you don't have to wait until then to show your kale pride: there are also T-shirts, with trendy slogans like "Powered by Kale" and "Highway to Kale." That's enough for us to set the alarm bells ringing.

- **Medjool dates:** It comes as a shock to include Medjool dates in a list of foods that encourage weight loss and promote health—especially when we tell you that Medjool dates contain a whopping 66 percent sugar. Sugar doesn't have any sirtuin-activating effects at all; instead, it has well-established connections to obesity, heart disease, and diabetes — just the reverse of what we're looking to do. Yet refined and replenished sugar is very different from sugar brought in a nature-borne vehicle supplemented with sirtuin-activating polyphenols: the date Medjool.

- **Parsley:** Parsley is a culinary conundrum. It so often occurs in recipes, but too often, it's the green token man. At best, we serve a pair of chopped sprigs and tossed as an afterthought on a plate, at worst a single sprig for decorative purposes only. This way, there on the plate, it is always languishing even after we have stopped feeding. This culinary style derives from its everyday use in ancient Rome as a garnish for eating after meals to restore breath, rather than being part of the meal itself. And what a shame, because parsley is a fantastic food that packs a vibrant, refreshing taste full of character.

- **Red endive:** Endive is a pretty new kid on the block in so far as vegetables go. Tale has it that a Belgian farmer invented endive in 1830 by mistake. The farmer stored chicory roots in his cellar and then used them as a type of coffee substitute, only to forget them. Upon his return, he discovered white leaves had sprouted, which he found to be tender, crunchy, and rather delicious upon degustation.

- **Red onions:** Since the time of our ancient ancestors, onions have been a culinary staple, being one of the first crops grown around 5,000 years ago. With such a long tradition of use and such strong health-giving properties, many civilizations that came before us have worshipped onions. They were held particularly by the Egyptians as objects of worship, seeing their circle-within-a-circle form as indicative of everlasting existence. The Greeks assumed onions made athletes better.

- **Red wine:** Any list of the top twenty Sirtfoods will not be complete without the inclusion of the original Sirtfood, red wine. The French phenomenon made headlines in the early 1990s, with it being revealed that with the French seeming to do something wrong with health (smoking, lack of fitness, and abundant food consumption), they had lower death rates from heart disease than countries like the United States.

- **Soy:** Soy products have a long tradition as an essential part of the diet of many countries in Asia-Pacific, such as China, Japan, and Korea. Researchers first turned on to soy after discovering that high soy-consuming countries had substantially lower rates of certain cancers, especially breast and prostate cancers. This is believed to be attributed to a specific category of polyphenols in soybeans known as isoflavones, which can favorably affect how estrogens function in the body, like daidzein and formononetin sirtuin-activators.

- **Strawberries:** In recent years, the fruit has been increasingly vilified, having a poor reputation in the rising enthusiasm for sugar. Luckily for berry lovers, such a malignant image couldn't be justified any worse. While all berries are powerhouses of nutrition, strawberries are earning their top twenty Sirtfood status due to their abundance of the fisetin sirtuin activator. And now studies support regular eating strawberries to promote healthy aging, staying off Alzheimer's, cancer, diabetes, heart disease, and osteoporosis. Its sugar content is minimal, a pure 31/2 ounces' tablespoon of sugar.

- **Turmeric:** Turmeric, a cousin of ginger, is the latest kid in food trends on the block, and Google calls it the ingredient of the 2015 breakout star. While we are just turning to it nowhere in the West, it has been valued for thousands of years in Asia, for both culinary and medical reasons. Incredibly, India is generating almost the entire world's turmeric stock, eating 80 percent of it.

- **Walnuts:** Dating back to 7000 BCE, walnuts are the oldest known human-made tree product, originating in ancient Persia, where they were the property of royalty. Fast forward to the modern-day, and walnuts are a success story in the US. California is leading the way, with California's Central Valley renowned for being the prime walnut-growing region. California walnuts provide the United States with 99 percent of commercial supply and staggering three-quarters worldwide walnut trade.

Beyond the Top Twenty Sirtfoods

Below we listed another forty foods that we discovered have Sirtfood properties too. They strongly urge you to add these foods to sustain and promote your weight reduction and health while you further broaden your diet collection.

Vegetables

- Broccoli.

- Bok choy/pak choi.

- Asparagus.

- Artichokes.

- Yellow endive.

- Watercress.

- White onions.

- Green beans.

- Shallots.

- Frisée.

Fruits

- Red grapes.

- Raspberries.

- Goji berries.

- Cranberries.

- Black plums.

- Black currants.

- Kumquats.

- Blackberries.

- Apples.

Nuts and Seeds

- Sunflower seeds.

- Pistachio nuts.

- Pecan nuts.

- Peanuts.

- Chia seeds.

- Chestnuts.

Grains and Pseudo-Grains

- Whole-wheat flour.

- Quinoa.

- Popcorn.

Beans

- White beans (e.g., cannellini or navy).

- Fava beans.

Herbs and Spices

- Ginger.

- Dried sage.

- Dried oregano.

- Dill (fresh and dried).

- Cinnamon.

- Chives.

- Peppermint (fresh and dried).

- Thyme (fresh and dried).

Beverages

- White tea.

- Black tea.

Chapter 6: How Many Sirtfoods Do You Need to Eat?

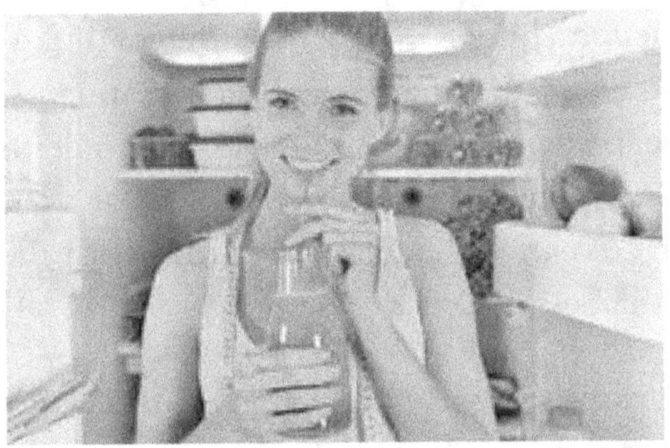

The Sirtfood Diet is separated into two fundamental stages (which are delineated in more prominent detail in the book):

To make Phase 1 as smooth sailing as possible, we will direct you one day at a time through the complete seven-day plan, including the lowdown on the Sirtfood green juice and easy-to-follow, delicious recipes at every stage. Phase 1 of the Sirtfood Diet is based on two distinct stages:

Days 1 to 3 are the most intensive, and during this time, you will consume up to a limit of 1,000 calories per day, consisting of:

- 3 x Sirtfood green juices.

- 1 x main meal.

Days 4 to 7 will see your daily consumption rise to a maximum of 1,500 calories, consisting of:

- 2 x Sirtfood green juices.

- 2 x main meals.

Ultimately, for sustained success, it's about tying it into the lifestyle and around daily life. But here are a few easy but big-impact tips to get the best result:

1. **Get a decent juicer:** Juicing is an integral part of the Sirtfood Diet and a juicer is one of the best investments you'll make for your wellbeing. Though the budget should be the deciding factor, some juicers are more efficient at extracting the juice from green leafy vegetables and herbs, with the Breville brand among the best juicers we've tried.

2. **Preparation is key:** One thing is evident from the abundance of feedback we've had: the most effective were those who prepared ahead of time. Get to know the ingredients and recipes and stock up on what's needed. You'll be surprised at how simple the whole process is with everything planned and ready.

3. **Save time:** Prepare cleverly when you're tight on time. Meals can be made the previous night. Juices can be made in bulk and stored in the refrigerator for up to three days (or longer in the freezer) until their sirtuin-activating nutrient levels begin to fall. Just shield it from light and add only when you're ready to eat it in the matcha.

4. **Eat early:** Eating earlier in the day is safer. Preferably, meals and juices should not be eaten later than 7 p.m. (To remember why to see page 71). Still, the diet is ideally built to suit your lifestyle, and late eaters often reap great benefits.

5. **Stretch out the juices:** They should be eaten at least one hour before or two hours after a meal to maximize the absorption of green juices and distributed throughout the day, rather than being too close together.

6. **Eat until satisfied:** Sirtfoods can have drastic effects on appetite, and some people will be complete before they nest. Listen to your body and feed until you are full rather than forcing down all food. Tell "Hara Hachi bu," as the long-lived Okinawans do, which loosely translates as "Eat until you're 80 percent full."

7. **Enjoy the ride:** Don't get stuck on the end goal, but remain conscious of the ride instead. This diet is about enjoying food in all its glory because of its health, but also for the joy and enjoyment it brings. Research indicates that we are much more likely to succeed if we keep our minds focused on the road rather than the final goal.

Now for the Phase 2

The key to success in this process is keeping your diet filled with Sirtfoods. To make it as simple as possible, we have prepared a seven-day menu plan for you to follow, including delicious family-friendly recipes, filled with Sirtfoods every day to the rafters (although see page 149 for children's advice). All you need to do is repeat the Seven Day Plan twice to complete Phase 2's fourteen days.

On each of the fourteen days, your diet will consist of:

- 3 x balanced sirtfood-rich meals.

- 1 x sirtfood green juice.

- 1 to 2 x optional snacks Sirtfood bite snacks.

Once again, when you have to consume these, there are no rigid rules. Be flexible throughout your day, and keep in mind two simple thumb rules are:

- Have your green juice either in the morning, at least 30 minutes before breakfast, or in the middle of the morning.

- Do your hardest to eat your dinner by 7 p.m.

Portion Sizes

During Phase 2, our attention is not on calorie counting. For the average person, this is not a practical approach or even a successful one over the long term. Alternatively, we concentrate on small servings, really well-balanced meals, and filling up on Sirtfoods so that you can continue to enjoy their fat-burning and health-promoting effects.

We've also designed the meals in the plan to make them satiate, making you feel satisfied for longer. That, combined with Sirtfoods' natural appetite-regulating effects, means you're not going to spend the next 14 days feeling hungry, but happily satisfied, well-fed, and extremely well-fed.

Just like in Phase 1, remember to listen and be guided by your appetite. If you make meals according to our instructions, and you are comfortably full before you have a meal, then stop eating is perfectly fine!

Chapter 7: Sirtuin Diet Plan

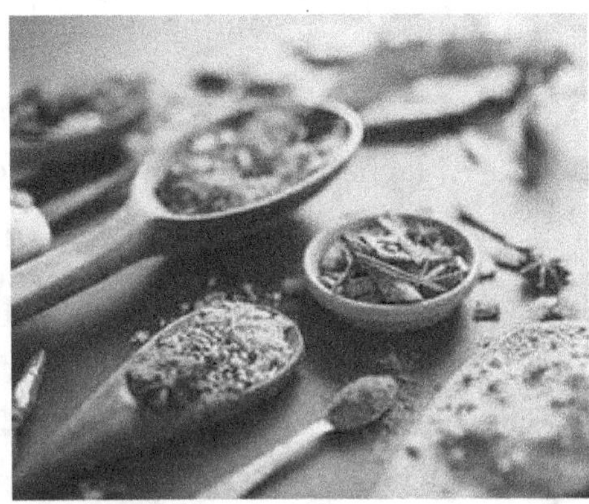

How you eat is your diet, restricting how you eat is dieting.

Before you will ever be successful at losing weight and maintaining your ideal size, you need to acknowledge the reality of where you are, get a firm and clear grasp on what it is you truly want, and then be honest with yourself about how you're going to make it happen.

The average American over-consumes solid fats and sugars, refined grains, sodium, and saturated fat. They also under-consume vegetables, fruits, whole grains, as well as the nationally recommended intake of dairy and oils.

If this sounds like it matches your current eating patterns, don't be too hard on yourself, you're certainly not alone. You've been practically brainwashed into adopting these poor nutrition habits.

The number of fast-food restaurants continues to grow, as do your options for pre-made, packaged foods full of empty calories and misleading promises.

When you live on a diet of foods devoid of all nutrition for too long, you find yourself getting sick and overweight. So, you turn to the following industry that profits from your poor health, the diet industry.

How many times have you found yourself dieting, starving yourself for weeks to lose 20 pounds? Maybe you've even been successful a time or two and lost weight, but within a few months, all the weight you lost had found its way home again and brought a few extra friends along.

Studies show that when you restrict your calories severely for an extended time, you will gain the weight back as quickly as it came off. You will do additional damage to your liver, kidneys, and muscle mass as well. Short-term calorie restriction, such as intermittent fasting or the first phase of the Sirtfood Diet, doesn't have the same effect as depleting your body of nutrition for 3 weeks or more (Muller, et al., 2015).

Dieting Does Not Work

More to the point, it's completely unnecessary, as we discovered earlier when we talked about traditional cultures and the Blue Zone of the world. They don't count calories or diet, and they live to be 100+ with their full physical and mental capacities until one night, they drift off into a peaceful, joyous slumber never to wake again. That sounds a lot better than spending the last few months, if not years, of your life in a hospital bed, unable to wash or feed yourself, let alone walk around or remember your grandchildren.

You get to choose your future, and it begins with choosing a healthy diet rich in delicious, fortifying, and age-defying sirtfoods.

When you're first starting to alter your diet, you may be wondering if taking supplements can help you integrate some sirtuin-activation benefits without actually changing the way you're eating. Can you just pop a pill that is full of blueberry extract or super greens?

The science is controversial on this subject, but any time you're trying to cheat your way to health, chances are you will end up cheating your health instead.

If your doctor or primary care physician has advised you to take a supplement, follow their advice. There are circumstances when supplementation is critical for your survival. There are many more circumstances when taking supplements is merely advisable. Vegans, for example, are almost always deficient in vitamin B12 and Omega-3 fatty acids because both nutrients are most commonly found in fatty, oily fish. If following an entirely plant-based diet is your ethical or moral choice, you may need to supplement for your best health.

But using supplements as a way to excuse poor dietary or lifestyle choices is never going to get you ahead in the game of life. Many studies suggest when specific vitamins, minerals, antioxidants or even polyphenols are isolated and consumed outside of their natural food source, they are not metabolized effectively and, in some cases, can even be detrimental to your health. Humans are very impressive in the field of science and medicine. Still, nature has secrets we haven't even begun to unravel, so whenever possible, it's in your best interest to find the most natural source of nutrition possible.

You may have first heard about the Sirtfood Diet because you saw a headline about Adele's miraculous weight loss. Or perhaps you heard scientists had discovered a "skinny gene" and the secret to accessing it was in this diet.

You want to lose weight, look great, and feel great in your skin.

That is a common and completely understandable desire, but it's not enough to get you the results you're dreaming of. At least not in the long-term. History has proven to us many times over that even if we succeed in reaching our goal weight, we're not satisfied. We return to our previous habits and the weight comes back.

One of the main reasons losing weight is ineffective is because it has an end or a result that you can achieve that allows you to give up. If you want a change in your life, you have to start with a change in your goals.

If you start looking deeper and making a commitment to your health, you'll find that there is never a moment that you permit yourself to stop. Even if you're relatively healthy today, you maintain a desire to stay healthy tomorrow and the following year, and 20 years from now. Health is a never-ending journey, and that is where your real success and results will lie. You won't have a deadline to abide by and you can't fail, as long as you're taking actions every day that are designed to improve some aspect of your health.

Sometimes you'll see and feel the results right away. The participants in the first Sirtfood Diet trial saw weight loss results within 7 days. But other times, the benefits are on a cellular level. You won't realize they're making such a difference in your life until you're 80 years old and the only one of your peers that have not been forced to move into assisted living.

One of the other significant reasons dieting has a less than impressive track record is because of the type of weight loss that is occurring.

The diseases associated with obesity aren't caused by excess weight. When you spend many years eating unhealthy foods, you damage your metabolic system and the hormones that support your metabolism. Issues like insulin and leptin resistance cause you to gain weight and develop even more lethal diseases, like diabetes and heart disease. The food you eat is the problem, and the weight is simply a by-product of a dysfunctional metabolic system.

If you heal the system by removing the foods that are damaging your hormones and adding foods that will heal and protect your entire body, the weight will come off naturally as a result of fixing the damage.

When you try to take the weight off through calorie restriction, excessive exercise or a combination of the two, you will likely lower the numbers on your scale. There is truth to the philosophy of "calories in, calories out." However, if you aren't considering the quality of the calories going in, you won't have any control over what comes off. You're just as likely to lose water weight and muscle mass as you are to lose any fat.

If you commit to providing your body with all the nutrition it needs to rebalance your hormones and protect your health, the weight you lose is going to be the weight you don't need: visceral fat around your vital organs and abdominal fat you've been struggling to get rid of for years. Your muscles will be protected, and your body will stay nicely hydrated.

Losing weight as a result of improved health is sustainable, so you must adjust your mindset and your goals if you truly want to be successful.

The best part about the Sirtfood Diet is that you can develop a plan specifically designed to suit your life and lifestyle. At the back of this book is are 2 appendices listing over 120 foods that would be ideal for you to enjoy any time of any day.

Do you have to eat them all? No, of course not. If you can't stand the taste of red onions, don't eat them. Add a little extra garlic to your dish instead, or just have another cup of green tea.

Are you limited to eating only these 120 plants for the rest of your life? Not! Foods that will activate your sirtuins are at the core of this diet, but they work best when they're complimenting a meal that is rounded out with healthy proteins and fats.

Many sirtfoods are probably already part of your standard eating plan, which may make you wonder why you're not healthier and trimmer now. The truth is, sirtfoods aren't miracle cures. Deep down, you know you have some bad habits that are hurting your health. Having strawberries on top of your ice cream, a mocha latte with an extra whip or the occasional garlic sauce in your take-out Chinese food does not qualify as a sirtfood rich diet, despite the presence of strawberries, coffee, and garlic.

Sirtfoods and quality proteins should be the majority of your diet, not an occasional sprinkle.

Instead of relying on processed sugar, experiment with the natural sugars in berries and other fruits, Medjool dates, and even the subtle sweetness of walnuts and other nuts. Trade-in meals doused with table salt for the uniquely salty tang of capers or the depth of savory flavors that can be found in a sauce made of garlic, onions, and red wine. Swap your bland vegetable oils for the richness of extra-virgin olive oil.

When you begin to experiment with the fantastic choices that are available to you, you will quickly realize that there are no limitations in the Sirtfood Diet. It is the way you used to eat that was limiting your enjoyment of food. It may take some time for your palette to adjust. Still, if you have patience and determination, you will be surprised how willingly your body will adapt to the new flavors that bring so much nutritional value.

You may also have to consider other factors in your lifestyle. If you're regularly eating on the run, you'll always be consuming your foods in a state of stress. This makes you more likely to eat faster, and therefore consume more calories than you need, and also make choices of convenience rather than a priority. When you take your time to eat, appreciating the value of the food, you will more satiated and less likely to overeat. Still, you will have to sacrifice something to make time in your day to appreciate your meals.

Also related to timing is making a conscious decision to eat earlier each day. When you consume more calories in the morning, you're fueling your body to perform all the necessary tasks of your day. When your hard work is over future use in the day, you don't need as much energy to support your relaxation hours. You certainly don't need the extra energy from a bag of chips or a complete drive-thru burger extra value meal an hour before you go to bed.

What it comes down to is the fact that the Sirtfood Diet is hugely flexible and variable; it will work in cooperation with your unique lifestyle. But you will still have to make some changes to your lifestyle that prioritize your health rather than your immediate gratification.

Chapter 8: Breakfasts Recipes

Strawberry Buckwheat Pancakes

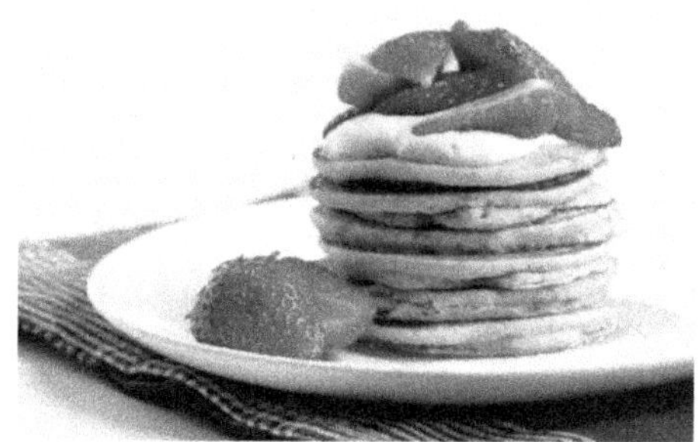

Preparation time: 15 minutes.

Cooking time: 30 minutes.

Servings: 4

Ingredients:

- 100 grams strawberries, chopped

- 100 grams buckwheat flour

- 1 egg

- 250 milliliters milk

- 2 teaspoons olive oil

- Freshly squeezed juice of 1 orange

Directions:

- Pour the milk into a bowl and mix in the egg and a teaspoon of olive oil.

- Stir the flour into the liquid mixture until smooth and creamy.

- Allow it to rest for 15 minutes.

- Heat a little oil in a pan and pour in a quarter of the mixture (or to the size you prefer).

- Sprinkle in a quarter of the strawberries into the batter.

- Cook for around 2 minutes on each side.

- Serve hot with a drizzle of orange juice.

Nutrition:

- **Calories:** 143

- **Total fat:** 3g

Sirtfood Mueslo

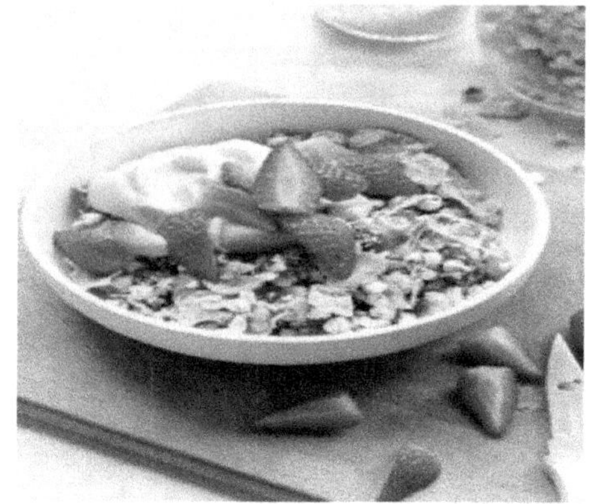

Preparation time: 5 minutes.

Cooking time: 10 minutes.

Servings: 1

Ingredients:

- 1 /4 cup (20 grams) buckwheat flakes

- 2 /3 cup (10 grams) buckwheat puffs

- 3 tablespoons (15 grams) coconut flakes or dried coconut

- 1 /4 cup (40 grams) Medjool dates, pitted and chopped

- 1 /8 cup (15 grams) walnuts, chopped

- 1(1 /2) tablespoon (10 grams) cocoa nibs

- 2 /3 cup (100 grams) strawberries, hulled and chopped

- 3 /8 cup (100 grams) plain Greek yogurt (or vegan alternative, such as soy or coconut yogurt)

Directions:

- Mix all the ingredients (leave out the strawberries and yogurt if not serving right away).

Nutrition:

- **Calories:** 515

- **Carbohydrates:** 76g

- **Fat:** 23g

- **Protein:** 37g

Strawberry and Nut Granola

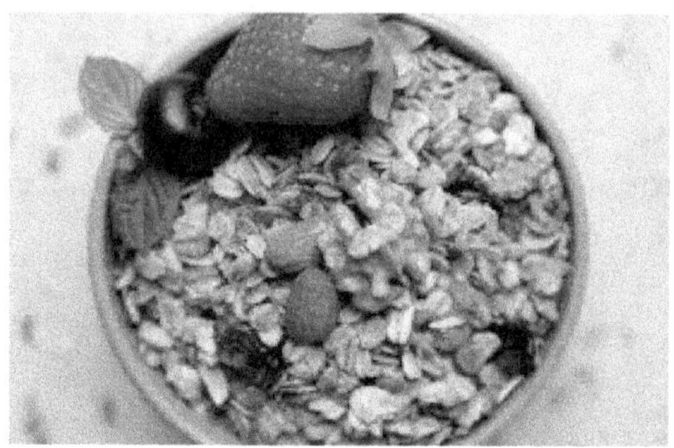

Preparation time: 20 minutes.

Cooking time: 1 hour.

Servings: 12

Ingredients:

- 200 grams (7 ounces) oats

- 250 grams (9 ounces) buckwheat flakes

- 100 grams (3(½) ounces) walnuts, chopped

- 100 grams (3(½) ounces) almonds, chopped

- 100 grams (3(½) ounces) dried strawberries

- 1½ teaspoon ground ginger

- 1½ teaspoon ground cinnamon

- 120 milliliters (4fl ounces) olive oil

- 2 tablespoons honey

Directions:

- Combine the oats, buckwheat flakes, nuts, ginger and cinnamon.

- In a saucepan, warm the oil and honey.

- Stir until the honey has melted.

- Pour the warm oil into the dry ingredients and mix well.

- Spread the mixture out on a large baking tray (or two) and bake in the oven at 150°C (300°F) for around 50 minutes until the granola is golden.

- Allow it to cool.

- Add in the dried berries.

- Store in an airtight container until ready to use.

Nutrition:

- **Calories:** 224

- **Carbohydrates:** 31.4g

- **Fat:** 8.2g

- **Protein:** 4.2g

Chilled Strawberry and Walnut Porridge

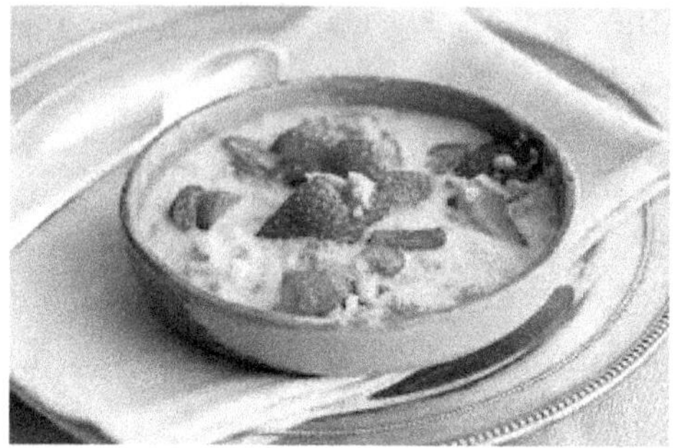

Preparation time: 10 minutes.

Cooking time: 15 minutes.

Servings: 1

Ingredients:

- 100 grams (3(½) ounces) strawberries

- 50 grams (2 ounces) rolled oats

- 4 walnut halves, chopped

- 1 teaspoon chia seeds

- 200 milliliters (7fl ounces) unsweetened soya milk

- 100 milliliters (3(½) ounces) water

Directions:

- Place the strawberries, oats, soya milk and water into a blender, and process until smooth.

- Stir in the chia seeds and mix well.

- Chill in the fridge overnight and serve in the morning with a sprinkling of chopped walnuts. It's simple and delicious.

Nutrition:

- **Calories:** 105

- **Protein:** 20g

- **Fat:** 3.4g

Fruit and Crunchy Nut Yogurt

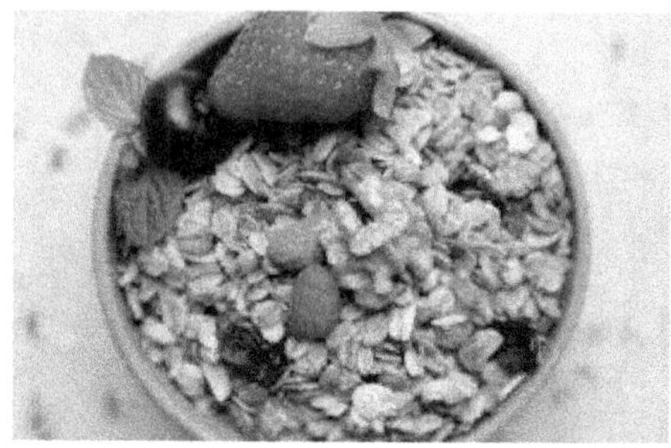

Preparation time: 15 minutes.

Cooking time: 10 minutes.

Servings: 1

Ingredients:

- 100 grams (3(½) ounces) plain Greek yogurt

- 50 grams (2 ounces) strawberries, chopped

- 6 walnut halves, chopped

- A Sprinkling of cocoa powder

Directions:

- Stir half of the chopped strawberries into the yogurt.

- Using a glass, place a layer of yogurt with a sprinkling of strawberries and walnuts, followed by another layer of the same until you reach the top of the glass.

- Garnish with walnuts pieces and a dusting of cocoa powder.

Nutrition:

- **Calories:** 200

- **Protein:** 26g

- **Fat:** 3.4g

Banana and Cinnamon Oatmeal

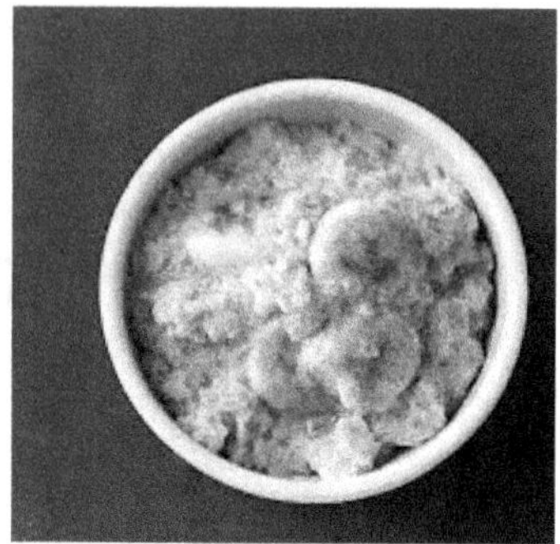

Preparation time: 10 minutes.

Cooking time: 5 minutes.

Servings: 6

Ingredients:

- 2 cups quick-cooking oats

- 4 cups fat-free milk

- 1 teaspoon ground cinnamon

- 2 chopped large ripe bananas

- 4 teaspoons brown sugar

- Extra ground cinnamon

Directions:

- Place milk in a skillet and bring to boil. Add oats and cook over medium heat until thickened for two to four minutes.

- Stir intermittently.

- Add cinnamon, brown sugar and banana, and stir to combine.

- If you want, serve with the extra cinnamon and milk. Enjoy!

Nutrition:

- **Calories** 208

- **Protein:** 27g

- **Fat:** 2.8g

Healthy Bagels

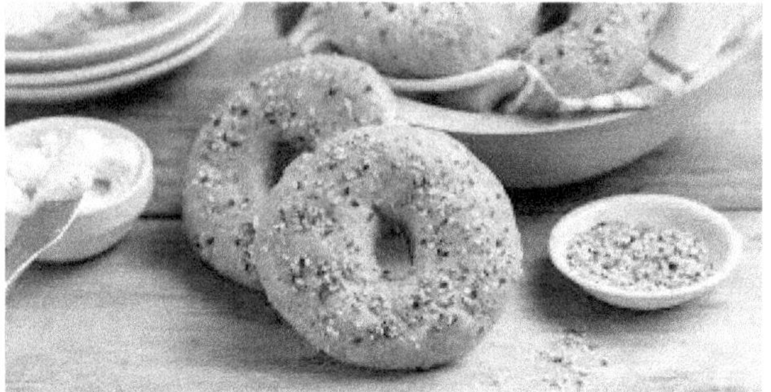

Preparation time: 30 minutes.

Cooking time: 1 hour.

Servings: 8

Ingredients:

- 1(½) cup warm water

- 1(¼) cup bread flour

- 2 tablespoons honey

- 2 cups whole-wheat flour

- 2 teaspoons yeast

- 1(½) tablespoon extra-virgin olive oil

- 1 tablespoon vinegar

Directions:

- In a bread machine, mix all the ingredients, and then process on dough cycle.

- Once done, create 8 pieces shaped like a flattened ball.

- Make a hole in the center of each ball using your thumb, then create a donut shape.

- In a greased baking sheet, place donut-shaped dough then covers and let it rise about ½ hour.

- Prepare about 2 inches of water to boil in a large pan.

- In boiling water, drop one at a time on the bagels and boil for 1 minute, then turn them once.

- Remove them and return to a baking sheet and bake at 350°F for about 20 to 25 minutes until golden brown.

Nutrition:

- **Calories:** 300

- **Protein:** 7.2g

- **Fat:** 3.5g

Cranberry and Orange Cereal

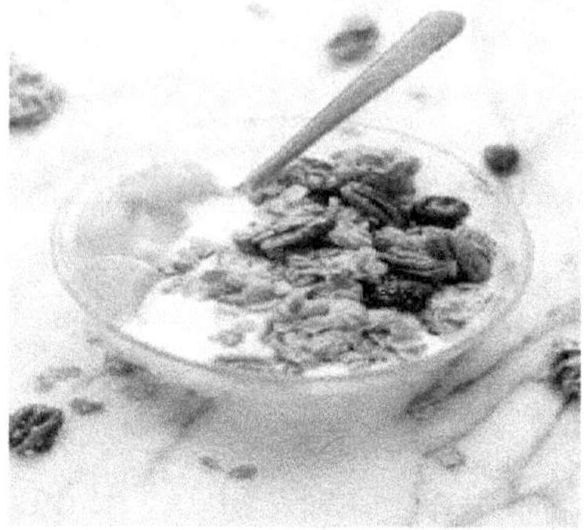

Preparation time: 10 minutes.

Cooking time: 5 minutes.

Servings: 1

Ingredients:

- ½ cup of water

- ½ cup of orange juice

- 1/3 cup of oat bran

- ¼ cup of dried cranberries

- Sugar

- Milk

Directions:

- In a bowl, combine all the ingredients.

- For about 2 minutes, microwave the bowl, then serve with sugar and milk.

Nutrition:

- **Calories:** 250

- **Protein:** 8.5g

- **Fat:** 4.2g

Vegan Rice Pudding

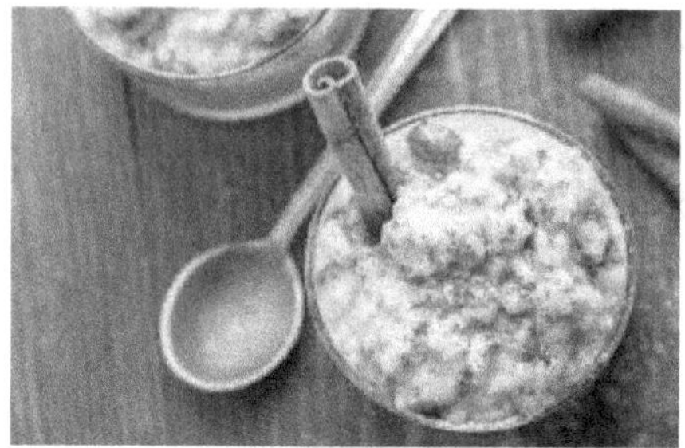

Preparation time: 10 minutes.

Cooking time: 5 minutes.

Servings: 8

Ingredients:

- ½ teaspoons ground cinnamon

- 1 cup rinsed basmati

- 1/8 teaspoon ground cardamom

- ¼ cup sugar

- 1/8 teaspoon pure almond extract

- 1-quart vanilla nondairy milk

- 1 teaspoon pure vanilla extract

Directions:

- Measure all the ingredients into a saucepan and stir well to combine.

- Bring to a boil over medium-high heat.

- Once boiling, reduce heat to low and simmer, stirring very frequently, about 15–20 minutes.

- Remove from heat and cold.

- Serve sprinkled with additional ground cinnamon if desired.

Nutrition:

- **Calories:** 350

- **Protein:** 6.5g

- **Fat:** 5g

Cinnamon Scented Quinoa Breakfast

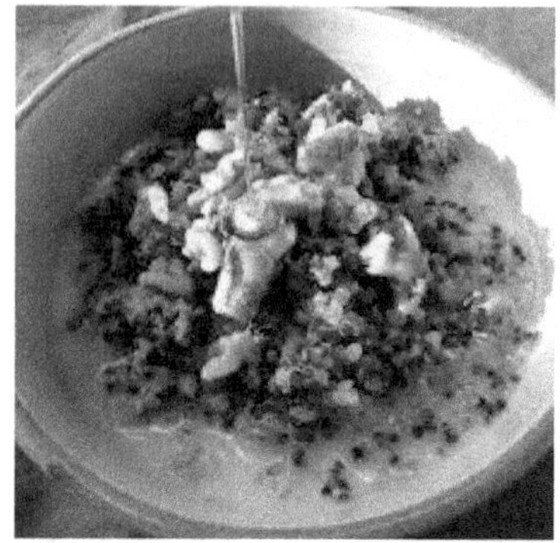

Preparation time: 15 minutes.

Cooking time: 20 minutes.

Servings: 4

Ingredients:

- Chopped walnuts for topping

- 1 ½ cup water

- Maple syrup for topping

- 2 cinnamon sticks

- 1 cup quinoa

Directions:

- Add the quinoa to a bowl and wash it in several changes of water until the water is clear.

- When washing quinoa, rub grains and allow them to settle before you pour off the water.

- Use a large fine-mesh sieve to drain the quinoa.

- Prepare your pressure cooker with a trivet and steaming basket.

- Place the quinoa and the cinnamon sticks in the basket and pour in the water.

- Close and lock the lid.

- Cook at high pressure for 6 minutes. When the cooking time is up, release the pressure using the quick-release method.

- Fluff the quinoa with a fork and remove the cinnamon sticks.

- Divide the cooked quinoa among serving bowls and top with maple syrup and chopped walnuts.

Nutrition:

- **Calories:** 550

- **Protein:** 35g

- **Fat:** 6g

Cheesy Baked Eggs

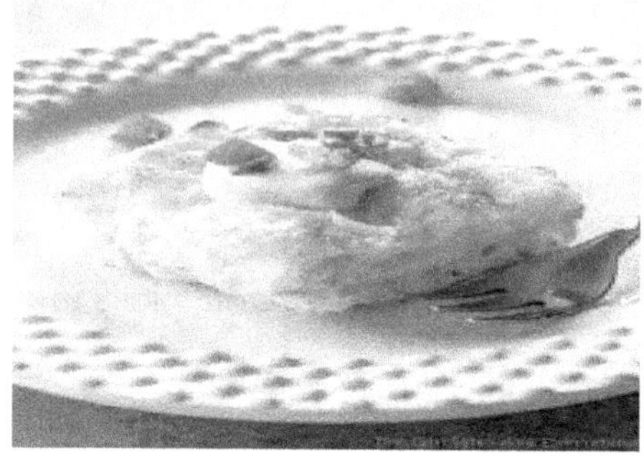

Preparation time: 20 minutes.

Cooking time: 30 minutes.

Servings: 4

Ingredients:

- 4 large eggs

- 75 grams (3 ounces) cheese, grated

- 25 grams (1 ounce) fresh rocket (arugula) leaves, finely chopped

- 1 tablespoon parsley

- ½ teaspoon ground turmeric

- 1 tablespoon olive oil

Directions:

- Grease each ramekin dish with a little olive oil.

- Divide the rocket (arugula) between the ramekin dishes, then break an egg into each one.

- Sprinkle a little parsley and turmeric on top, then sprinkle on the cheese.

- Place the ramekins in a preheated oven at 220°C/425°F for 15 minutes until the eggs are set and the cheese is bubbling.

Nutrition:

- **Calories:** 450

- **Protein:** 26g

- **Fat:** 4g

Oatmeal Banana Pancakes with Walnuts

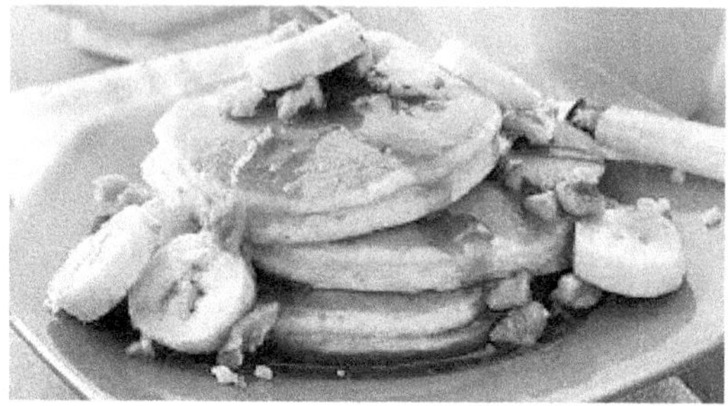

Preparation time: 15 minutes.

Cooking time: 20 minutes.

Servings: 8

Ingredients:

- 1 finely diced firm banana

- 1 cup whole-wheat pancake mix

- 1/8 cup chopped walnuts

- ¼ cup old-fashioned oats

Directions:

- Make the pancake mix according to the directions on the package.

- Add walnuts, oats, and chopped banana.

- Coat a skillet with cooking spray.

- Add about ¼ cup of the pancake batter onto the griddle when hot.

- Turn pancake over when bubbles form on top. Cook until golden brown.

- Serve immediately.

Nutrition:

- **Calories:** 425

- **Protein:** 23g

- **Fat:** 3.7g

Green Laden Egg Scramble

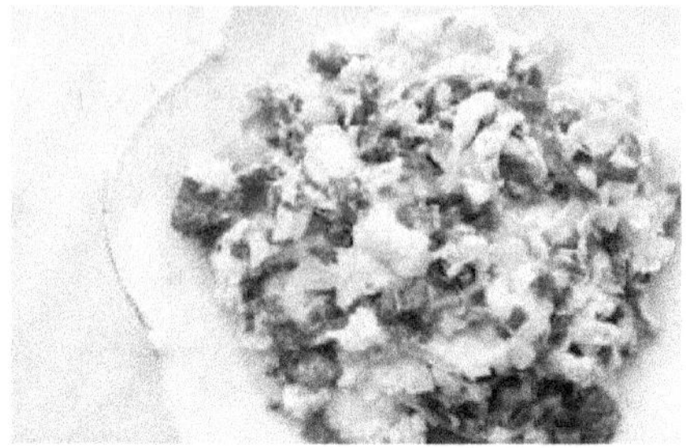

Preparation time: 5 minutes.

Cooking time: 10 minutes.

Servings: 1

Ingredients:

- 2 eggs, whisked

- 25 grams (1 ounce) rocket (arugula) leaves

- 1 teaspoon chives, chopped

- 1 teaspoon fresh basil, chopped

- 1 teaspoon fresh parsley, chopped

- 1 tablespoon olive oil

Directions:

- Mix the eggs with the rocket (arugula) and herbs.

- Heat the oil in a frying pan and pour it into the egg mixture.

- Gently stir until it's lightly scrambled.

- Season and serve.

Nutrition:

- **Calories:** 350

- **Protein:** 20g

- **Fat:** 3.2g

Spicy Scramble

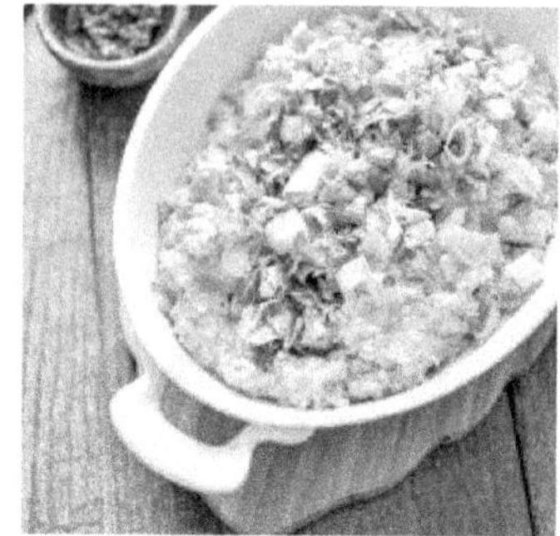

Preparation time: 5 minutes.

Cooking time: 10 minutes.

Servings: 1

Ingredients:

- 25 grams (1 ounce) kale, finely chopped

- 2 eggs

- 1 spring onion (scallion) finely chopped

- 1 teaspoon turmeric

- 1 tablespoon olive oil

- Sea salt to taste

- Freshly ground black pepper to taste

Directions:

- Crack the eggs into a bowl.

- Add the turmeric and whisk them.

- Season with salt and pepper.

- Heat the oil in a frying pan, add the kale and spring onions (scallions) and cook until it has wilted.

- Pour in the beaten eggs and stir until eggs have scrambled together with the kale.

Nutrition:

- **Calories:** 355

- **Protein:** 22g

- **Fat:** 3.6g

Sweet Potato Breakfast

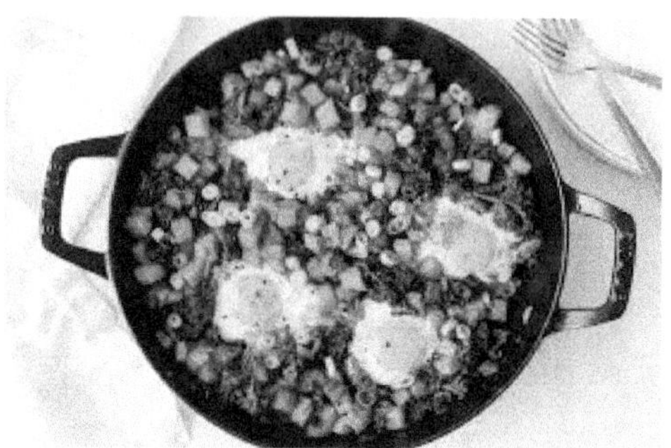

Preparation time: 10 minutes.

Cooking time: 15 minutes.

Servings: 2

Ingredients:

- 1 tablespoon maple syrup

- ¼ cup fat-free coconut Greek yogurt

- 1/8 cup unsweetened toasted coconut flakes

- 1 chopped apple

- Potatoes

Directions:

- Preheat oven to 400°F.

- Place your potatoes on a baking sheet.

- Bake them for 45–60 minutes or until soft.

- Use a sharp knife to mark "X" on the potatoes and fluff pulp with a fork.

- Top with coconut flakes, chopped apple, Greek yogurt, and maple syrup.

- Serve immediately.

Nutrition:

- **Calories:** 375

- **Protein:** 27g

- **Fat:** 4.2g

French Toast with Apple Sauce

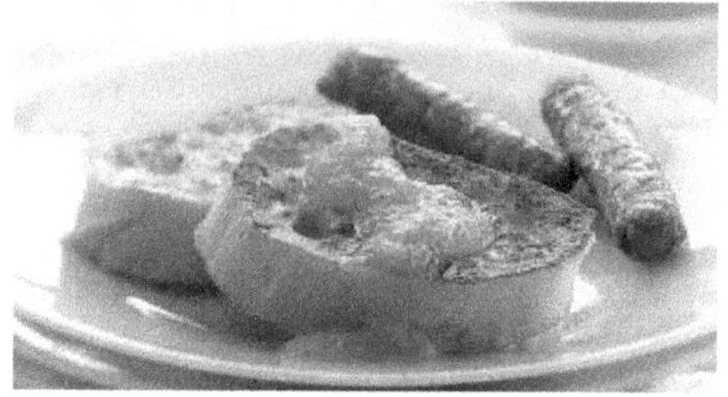

Preparation time: 5 minutes.

Cooking time: 10 minutes.

Servings: 6

Ingredients:

- ¼ cup unsweetened applesauce

- ½ cup skim milk

- 2 packets of Stevia

- 2 eggs

- 6 slices whole-wheat bread

- 1 teaspoon ground cinnamon

Directions:

- Mix well applesauce, sugar, cinnamon, milk, and eggs in a mixing bowl.

- One slice at a time, soak the bread into an applesauce mixture until wet.

- On medium fire, heat a large nonstick skillet.

- Add soaked bread on one side and another on the other side. Cook in a single layer in batches for 2–3 minutes per side on medium-low fire or until lightly browned.

- Serve and enjoy.

Nutrition:

- **Calories:** 380

- **Protein:** 25g

- **Fat:** 3.8g

Chapter 9: Juices and Smoothies

Kale Kiwi Smoothie

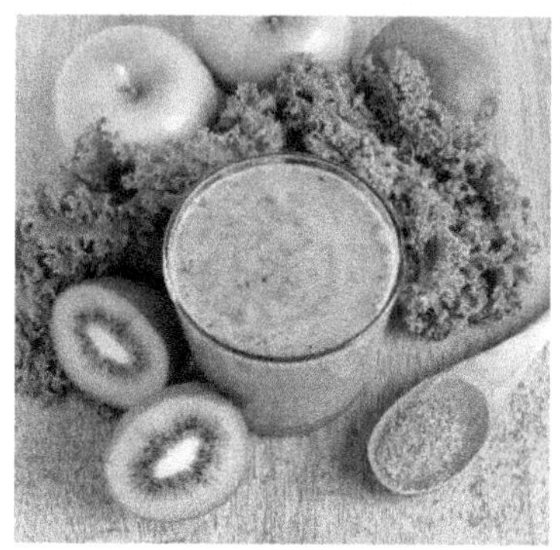

Preparation time: 10 minutes.

Cooking time: 5 minutes.

Servings: 1

Ingredients:

- 1 cup kale, chopped

- 2 apples

- 3 kiwis

- 1 tablespoon flax seeds

- 1 tablespoon royal jelly

- 1 cup crushed ice

Directions:

- Place all the ingredients into a blender and cover them with water. Blitz until smooth. You can also add some crushed ice and a mint leaf to garnish.

Nutrition:

- **Calories:** 146

Salad Smoothie

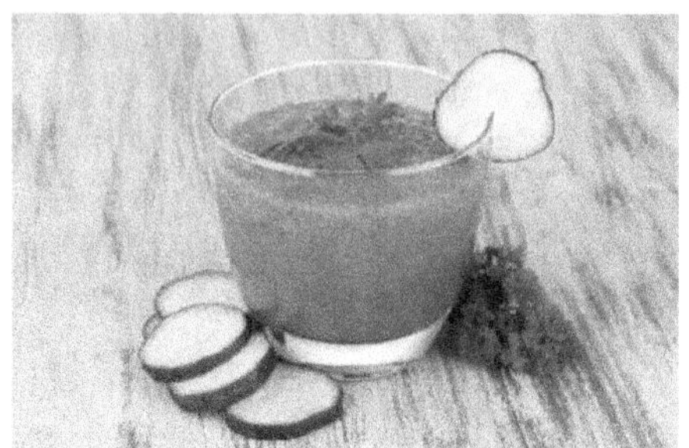

Preparation time: 10 minutes.

Cooking time: 5 minutes.

Servings: 1

Ingredients:

- 1 cup arugula

- ½ cucumber

- 1/2 small red onion

- 2 tablespoons parsley

- 2 tablespoons lemon juice

- 1 cup crushed ice

- 1 tablespoon olive oil or cumin oil

Directions:

- Put all the ingredients into a blender with some water and blitz until smooth. Add ice to make your smoothie refreshing.

Nutrition:

- **Calories:** 105

Avocado Kale Smoothie

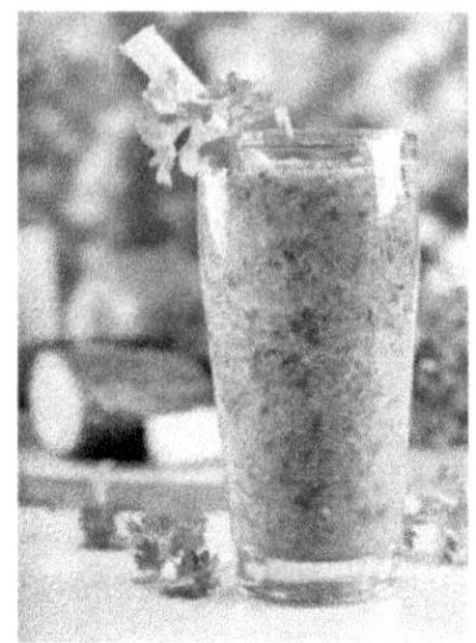

Preparation time: 10 minutes.

Cooking time: 5 minutes.

Servings: 1

Ingredients:

- 1 cup kale

- ½ avocado

- 1 cup cucumber

- 1 celery stalk

- 1 tablespoon chia seeds

- 1 cup crushed ice

- 1 tablespoon spirulina

Directions:

- Place all the ingredients into a blender and add in enough water to cover them. Process until smooth, serve and enjoy.

Nutrition:

- **Calories:** 156

Kale Banana Apple Smoothie

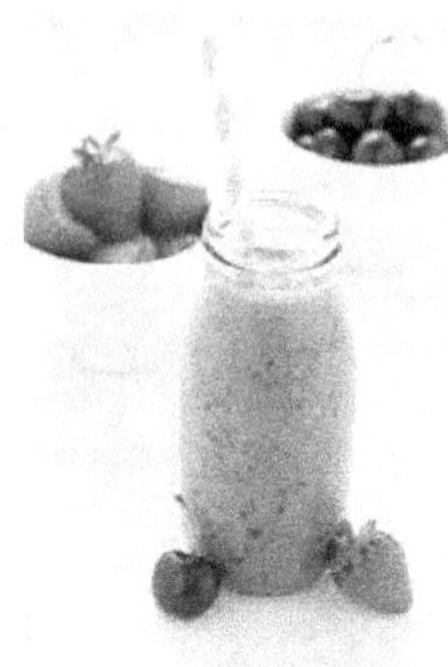

Preparation time: 10 minutes.

Cooking time: 5 minutes.

Servings: 1

Ingredients:

- 1 cup kale

- 2 apples

- 3/4 avocado

- 1 banana

- 1 cup crushed ice

Directions:

- Place all the ingredients into a blender and process until smooth. Serve and enjoy.

Nutrition:

- **Calories:** 132

Kale Cucumber Apple Smoothie

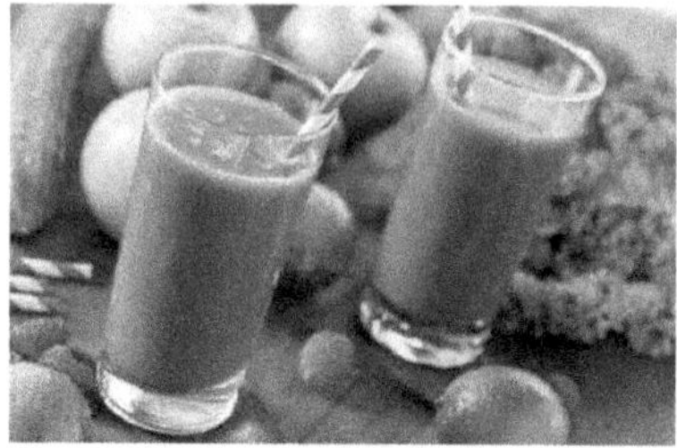

Preparation time: 10 minutes.

Cooking time: 5 minutes.

Servings: 1

Ingredients:

- 1 cup kale

- 2 apples

- 1 avocado

- 1 lime

- 1/4 cup raspberries

- 1 cucumber

- 1 cup crushed ice

Directions:

- Place all the ingredients into the blender with enough water to cover them and blitz until smooth.

Nutrition:

- **Calories:** 77

Grapefruit Kale Smoothie

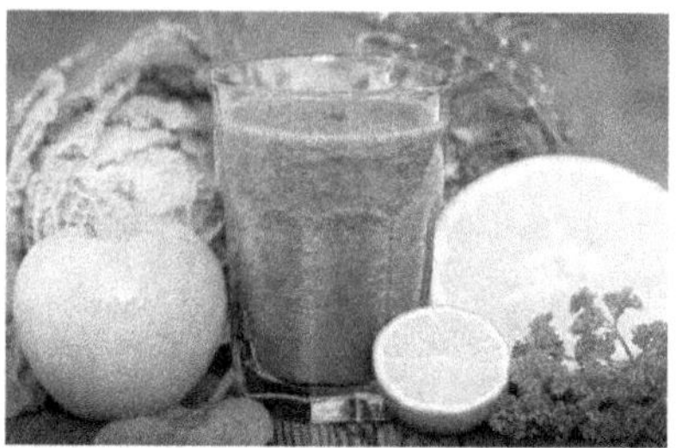

Preparation time: 10 minutes.

Cooking time: 5 minutes.

Servings: 1

Ingredients:

- 1 large grapefruit

- 1 apple

- 1 cup watercress

- 2 kale leaves

- 1 tablespoon dill (optional)

- 1 cup crushed ice

Directions:

- Place all the ingredients into a blender and add enough water to cover them. Process until creamy and smooth.

Nutrition:

- **Calories:** 306

Pear Cilantro Smoothie

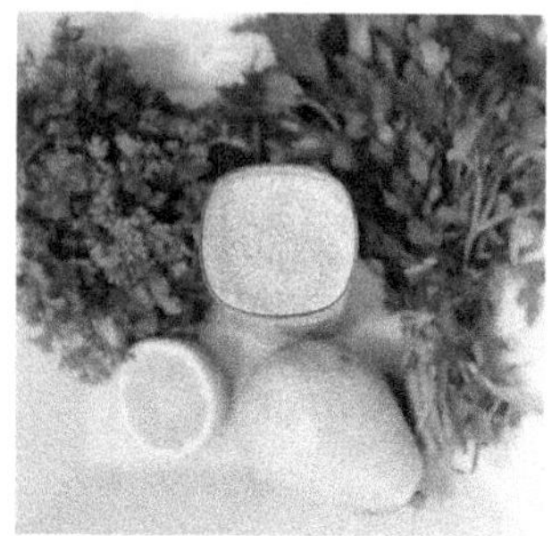

Preparation time: 10 minutes.

Cooking time: 5 minutes.

Servings: 1

Ingredients:

- 1 cup parsley leaves

- 1 pear

- 3/4 avocado

- ½ lemon—juice

- 1 tablespoon chopped cilantro

- 1 cup crushed ice

Directions:

- Place all the ingredients into a blender with enough water to cover them and process until smooth. Add a few ice cubes and enjoy.

Nutrition:

- **Calories:** 369

Kale Avocado Smoothie

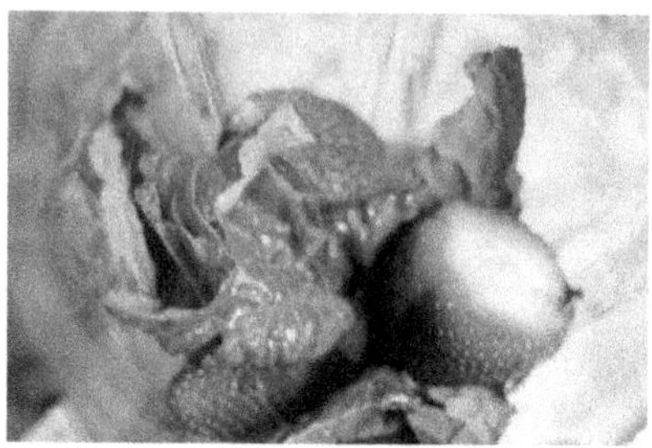

Preparation time: 10 minutes.

Cooking time: 5 minutes.

Servings: 1

Ingredients:

- 1 cup strawberries

- 1 cup kale

- 1/2 avocado

- 1/2 lemon

- 1 cup crushed ice

Directions:

- Place all the ingredients into a blender with enough water to cover them and process until smooth. Add a few ice cubes and enjoy.

Nutrition:

- **Calories:** 340

Kale, Parsley, and Banana Smoothie

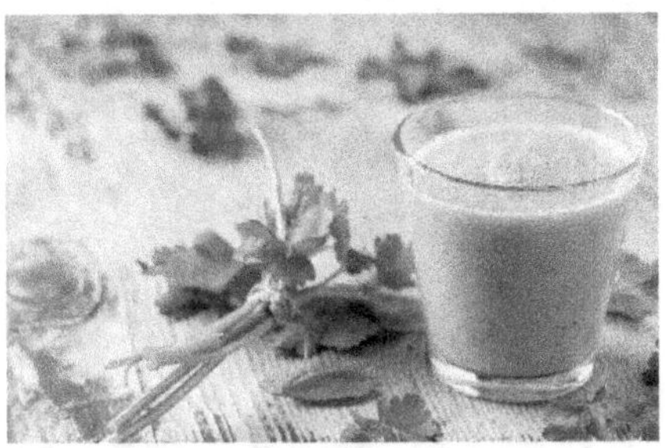

Preparation time: 10 minutes.

Cooking time: 5 minutes.

Servings: 1

Ingredients:

- 1 cup chopped kale

- 2 bananas

- ½ cup chopped parsley

- 1 cup crushed ice

Directions:

- Place all the ingredients into a blender with enough water to cover them and process until smooth. Add a few ice cubes and enjoy.

Nutrition:

- **Calories:** 335

Kefir Kale Banana Orange Chia Smoothie

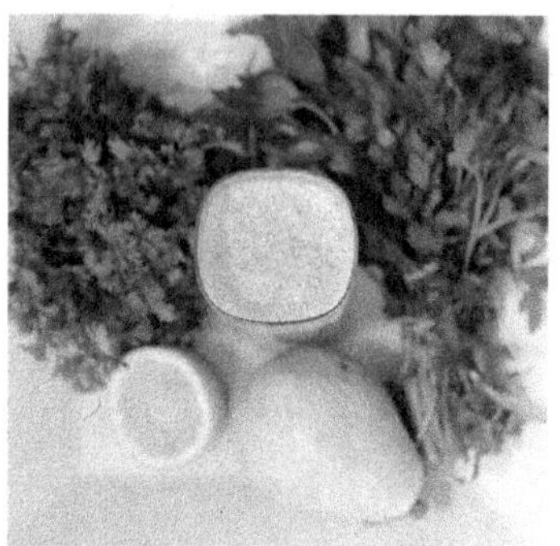

Preparation time: 10 minutes.

Cooking time: 5 minutes.

Servings: 1

Ingredients:

- 1/2 orange

- 1 banana

- 1 cup kale

- 1/4 cup chia seeds

- 1/2 cup kefir

- 1 cup crushed ice

Directions:

- Place all the ingredients into a blender with enough water to cover them and process until smooth. Add a few ice cubes and enjoy.

Nutrition:

- **Calories:** 345

Chapter 10: Phase 1 Recipes

Chocolate Waffles

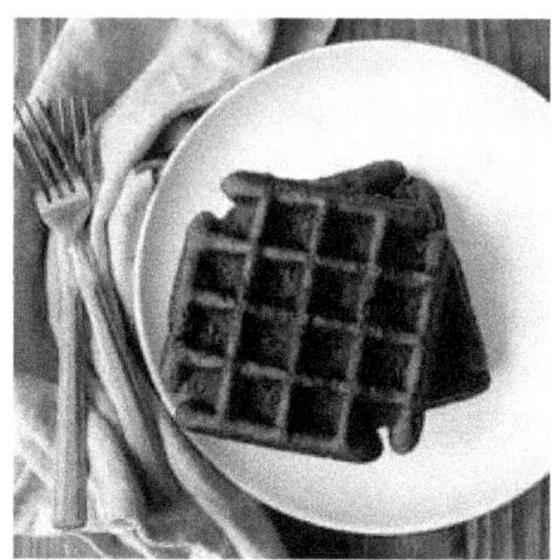

Preparation time: 15 minutes.

Cooking time: 24 minutes.

Servings: 8

Ingredients:

- 2 cups unsweetened almond milk

- 1 tablespoon fresh lemon juice

- 1 cup buckwheat flour

- ½ cup cacao powder

- ¼ cup flaxseed meal

- 1 teaspoon baking soda

- 1 teaspoon baking powder

- ¼ teaspoon kosher salt

- 2 large eggs

- ½ cup coconut oil, melted

- ¼ cup dark brown sugar

- 2 teaspoons vanilla extract

- 2 ounces unsweetened dark chocolate, chopped roughly

Directions:

- In a bowl, add the almond milk and lemon juice and mix well.

- Set aside for about 10 minutes.

- In a bowl, place buckwheat flour, cacao powder, flaxseed meal, baking soda, baking powder and salt and mix well.

- In the bowl of the almond milk mixture, place the eggs, coconut oil, brown sugar and vanilla extract and beat until smooth.

- Now, place the flour mixture and beat until smooth.

- Gently, fold in the chocolate pieces.

- Preheat the waffle iron and then grease it.

- Place the desired amount of the mixture into the preheated waffle iron and cook for about 3 minutes or until golden brown.

- Repeat with the remaining mixture.

- Serve warm.

Nutrition:

- **Calories**: 295

Salmon & Kale Omelet

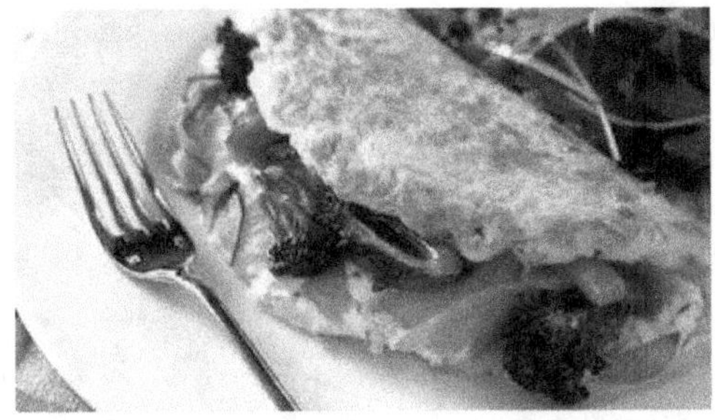

Preparation time: 10 minutes.

Cooking time: 7 minutes.

Servings: 4

Ingredients:

- 6 eggs

- 2 tablespoons unsweetened almond milk

- Salt and ground black pepper, as required

- 2 tablespoons olive oil

- 4 ounces smoked salmon, cut into bite-sized chunks

- 2 cup fresh kale, tough ribs removed and chopped finely

- 4 scallions, chopped finely

Directions:

- In a bowl, place the eggs, coconut milk, salt and black pepper and beat well. Set aside.

- In a nonstick wok, heat the oil over medium heat.

- Place the egg mixture evenly and cook for about 30 seconds, without stirring.

- Place the salmon kale and scallions on top of the egg mixture evenly.

- Now, adjust the heat to low and cook, covered for about 4–5 minutes or until the omelet is done completely.

- Uncover the wok and cook for about 1 minute.

- Carefully, transfer the omelet onto a serving plate and serve.

Nutrition:

- **Calories**: 210

Strawberry, Apple & Arugula Salad

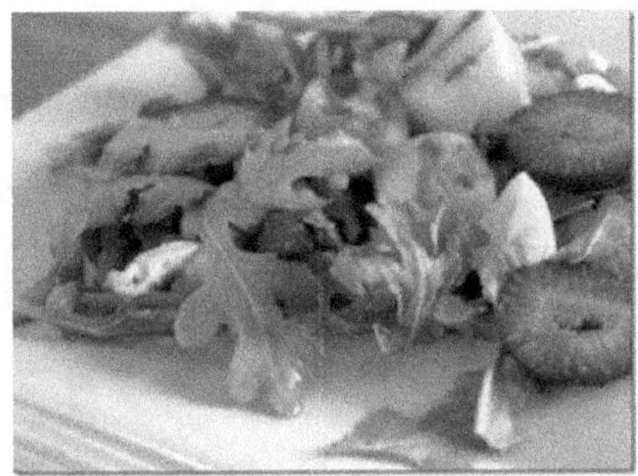

Preparation time: 15 minutes.

Cooking time: 0 minutes.

Servings: 4

Ingredients:

For the salad:

- 4 cups fresh baby arugula

- 2 apples, cored and sliced

- 1 cup fresh strawberries, hulled and sliced

- ¼ cup walnuts, chopped

- 4 tablespoons olive oil

- Salt and ground black pepper, as required

Directions:

- For the salad, place all the ingredients in a large bowl and mix well.

- For the dressing, place all the ingredients in a bowl and beat until well combined.

- Pour the dressing over the salad and toss it all to coat thoroughly.

- Serve immediately.

Nutrition:

- **Calories:** 243

Raspberry & Kale Salad

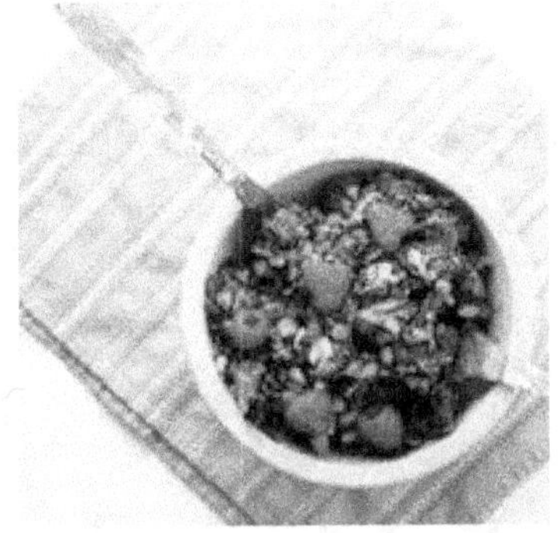

Preparation time: 15 minutes.

Cooking time: 0 minutes.

Servings: 2

Ingredients:

For the salad:

- 3 cups fresh baby kale

- ½ cup fresh raspberries

- ¼ cup walnuts, chopped

For the dressing:

- 1 tablespoon extra-virgin olive oil

- 1 tablespoon apple cider vinegar

- ½ teaspoon pure maple syrup

- Salt and ground black pepper, as required

Directions:

- **For the salad:** in a salad bowl, place all the ingredients and mix.

- **For the dressing:** place all the ingredients in another bowl and beat until well combined.

- Place dressing on top of the salad and toss to coat thoroughly.

- Serve immediately.

Nutrition:

- **Calories:** 228

Cucumber & Onion Salad

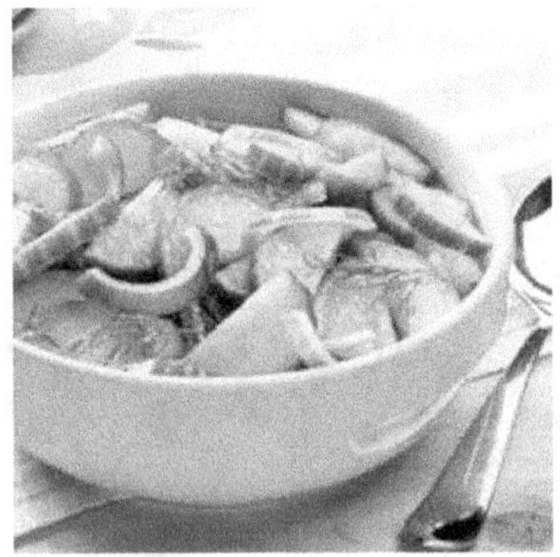

Preparation time: 10 minutes.

Cooking time: 0 minutes.

Servings: 4

Ingredients:

- 3 large cucumbers, sliced thinly

- ½ cup red onion, sliced

- 2 tablespoons olive oil

- 1 tablespoon fresh apple cider vinegar

- Sea salt, to taste

- ¼ cup fresh parsley, chopped

Directions:

- In a salad bowl, place all the ingredients and toss to coat thoroughly.

- Serve immediately.

Nutrition:

- **Calories:** 81

Shrimp Salad

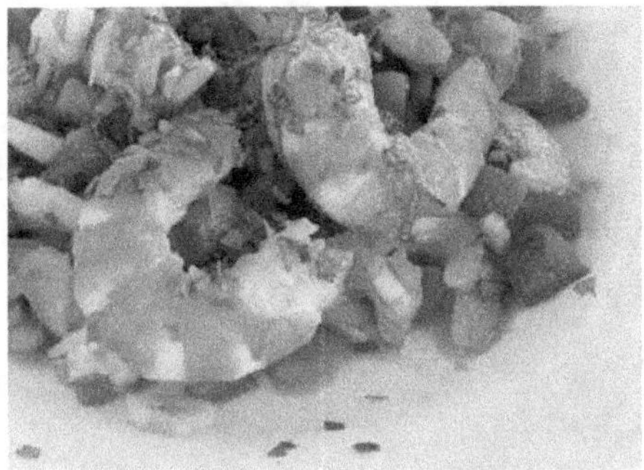

Preparation time: 15 minutes.

Cooking time: 6 minutes.

Servings: 6

Ingredients:

For the shrimp:

- 1 tablespoon olive oil

- 1 garlic clove, crushed

- 2 tablespoons fresh rosemary, chopped

- 1-pound raw shrimp, peeled and deveined

- ¼ teaspoon red pepper flakes, crushed

- Salt and ground black pepper, as required

For the salad:

- 8 cups fresh arugula

- 3 tablespoons olive oil

- 2 tablespoons fresh lime juice

- Salt and ground black pepper, as required

Directions:

- In a large wok, heat oil over medium heat and sauté 1 garlic clove for about 1 minute.

- Add the shrimp with red pepper flakes, salt and black pepper and cook for about 4–5 minutes.

- Remove the wok of shrimp from heat and set aside to cool.

- In a large bowl, add the shrimp, arugula, oil, lime juice, salt and black pepper and gently toss to coat.

- Serve immediately.

Nutrition:

- **Calories:** 182

Buckwheat Burgers

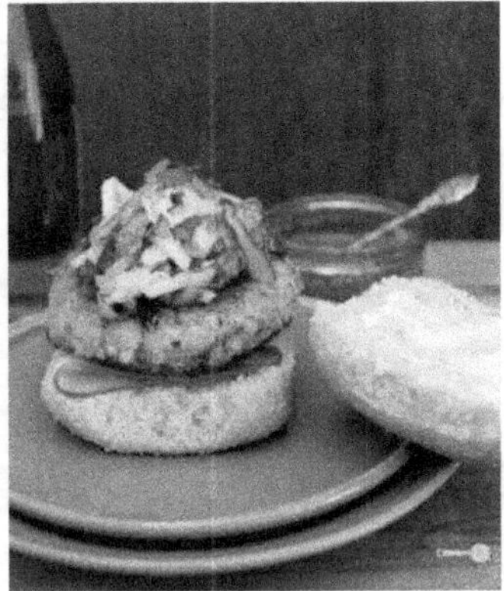

Preparation time: 20 minutes.

Cooking time: 1(¼) hours.

Servings: 4

Ingredients:

For the patties:

- ¾ cup dry buckwheat

- 1(½) cups water

- Salt, as required

- 2 tablespoons olive oil, divided

- ½ of large red onion, chopped finely

- ½ of a large carrot, peeled and grated

- ½ of celery stalk, chopped finely

- 1 fresh kale leaf, tough ribs removed, and chopped finely

- 1 large cooked sweet potato, mashed

- 2 tablespoons almond butter

- 2 tablespoons low-sodium soy sauce

For serving:

- 6 cups fresh baby kale

- 2 cups cherry tomatoes, halved

- Tomatoes

- Cabbage

Directions:

- Preheat your oven to 350°F.

- Line a baking sheet with parchment paper.

- **For the patties:** Heat a nonstick frying pan over medium heat and toast the buckwheat for about 5–6 minutes, stirring continuously.

- Add the water and salt and bring to a boil over high heat.

- Adjust the heat to low and cook, covered for about 15 minutes or until all the water is absorbed.

- Meanwhile, put 1 tablespoon of the oil over medium heat and sauté the onion for about 4–5 minutes.

- Add the carrot and celery and cook for about 5 minutes.

- Stir in the remaining ingredients and remove from the heat.

- Transfer the mixture into a bowl with buckwheat and stir to combine.

- Set aside to cool completely.

- Make 4 equal-sized patties from the mixture.

- Arrange the patties onto the prepared baking sheet in a single layer and bake for about

- Bake for approximately 20 minutes per side.

- Divide the greens, tomatoes, cabbage, and bell pepper onto serving plates.

- Top each plate with 1 patty and serve

Nutrition:

- **Calories:** 340

Kale with Pine Nuts

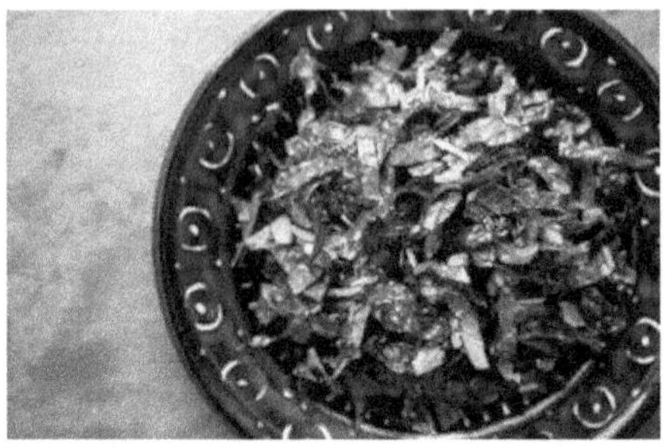

Preparation time: 10 minutes.

Cooking time: 10 minutes.

Servings: 4

Ingredients:

- 1 tablespoon olive oil

- 2 garlic cloves, minced

- 1(½) pounds fresh kale, tough ribs removed and chopped

- ¼ cup water

- 3 teaspoons red wine vinegar

- Salt and ground black pepper, as required

- 2 tablespoons pine nuts

Directions:

- Heat the olive oil in a large wok over medium heat and sauté the garlic for about 1 minute.

- Add kale and cook for about 3–4 minutes.

- Add the water, vinegar, salt and black pepper and cook for 4–5 minutes.

- Remove from heat and stir in the pine nuts.

- Serve immediately.

Nutrition:

- **Calories:** 146

Sautéed Mushrooms

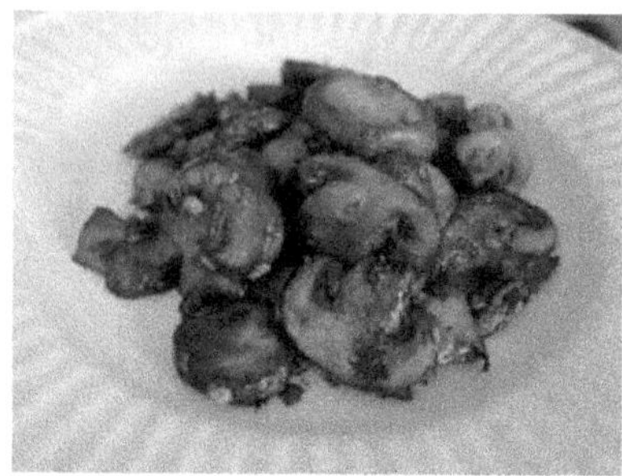

Preparation time: 10 minutes.

Cooking time: 15 minutes.

Servings: 2

Ingredients:

- 2 tablespoons olive oil

- 2–3 tablespoons red onion, minced

- ½ teaspoon garlic, minced

- 12 ounces fresh mushrooms, sliced

- 1 tablespoon fresh parsley

- 1 teaspoon fresh lemon juice

- Salt and ground black pepper, to taste

Directions:

- In a sauté pan, heat the oil over medium heat and sauté the onion and garlic for 3–4 minutes.

- Add the mushrooms and cook for 8–10 minutes or until desired doneness.

- Stir in the parsley, lemon juice, salt and black pepper and remove from the heat.

- Serve hot.

Nutrition:

- **Calories** 163

Chocolate Bites

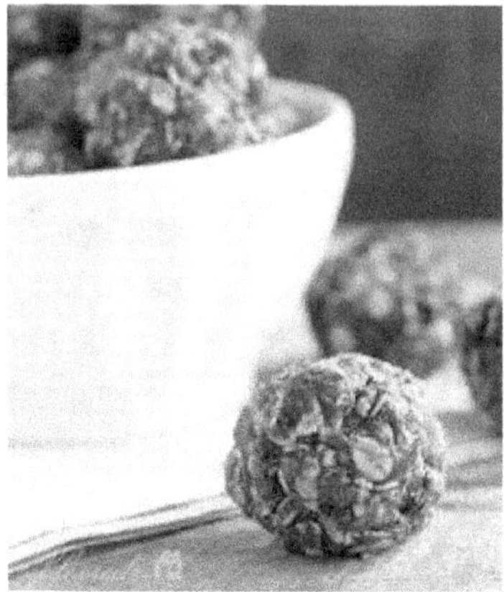

Preparation time: 15 minutes.

Cooking time: 0 minutes.

Servings: 15

Ingredients:

- 1 cup dates, pitted

- 2/3 cup gluten-free, rolled oats

- ¼ cup unsweetened dark chocolate, chopped roughly

- 1 tablespoon chia seeds

- 3 tablespoons almond butter

- ½ cup cacao powder

Directions:

- In a food processor, place dates and pulse until finely chopped.

- Add the remaining ingredients except for cacao powder and pulse until just combined.

- Make 1-ich balls from the mixture.

- In a shallow plate, place the cacao powder.

- Coat the balls with cacao powder and arrange them onto a parchment paper-lined baking sheet.

- Freeze for 15 minutes or until set altogether before serving.

Nutrition:

- **Calories:** 104

Chapter 11: Phase 2 Recipes

Chicken with Red Onion and Kale

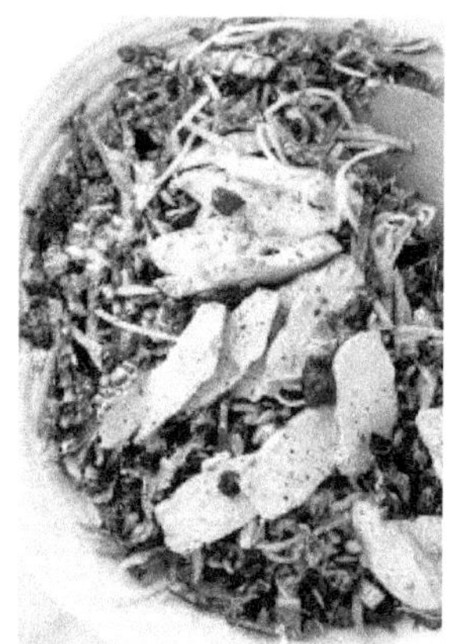

Preparation time: 30 minutes.

Cooking time: 20 minutes.

Servings: 3

Ingredients:

- 120 grams chicken breast

- 130 grams of tomatoes

- 1 bird's-eye chili

- 1 tablespoon of capers

- 5 grams of parsley

- Juice of half a lemon

- 2 teaspoons of extra-virgin olive oil

- 2 teaspoons of turmeric

- 50 grams of curly kale

- 20 grams of red onion

- 1 teaspoon fresh ginger

- 50 grams of buckwheat

Directions:

- Marinate the chicken breast for 10 minutes with 1/4 of lemon juice, 1 teaspoon of extra-virgin olive oil, and 1 teaspoon of turmeric powder.

- Cut 130 grams of tomatoes into chunks, remove the inside, season with the chili pepper, 1 tablespoon of capers, 1 teaspoon of turmeric and one of extra-virgin olive oil, 1/4 lemon juice, and 5 grams of chopped parsley.

- Cook the drained chicken breast on high heat for one minute per side and then put it in the oven for about 10 minutes at 220°F. Let it rest covered by aluminum foil. Steam the minced curly kale for 5 minutes, in a pan, fry the red onion, a teaspoon of grated fresh ginger, and a teaspoon of extra-virgin olive oil; add the boiled cabbage and leave to flavor for one minute on the fire, boil the buckwheat with turmeric, drain and serve with the chicken, tomatoes and chopped cabbage.

Nutrition:

- **Calories** 550

Pan-Fried Chicken, Banana, and Kale

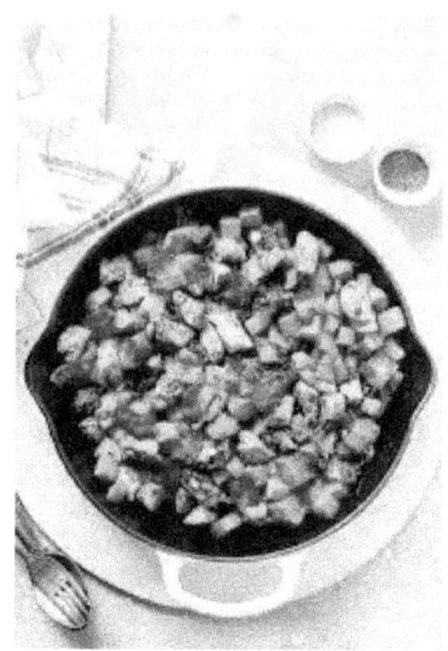

Preparation time: 30 minutes.

Cooking time: 20 minutes.

Servings: 3

Ingredients:

- 4 banana (medium)

- 300 grams kale

- 400 grams chicken breast

- 1 Tropea red onions

- 1 clove garlic

- 1 glass of dry white wine

- Salt to taste

Directions:

- We carefully clean the banana by washing them very carefully without peeling them: most of the trace elements of this rhizome are in the skin and it is a pity to eliminate them because many of its precious virtues would be lost.

- After washing them, cut them into cubes of about 2 centimeters on each side and dip them in cold water. We wash and dry the kale carefully and cut it into strips. We cut the chicken breast into cubes and dry it carefully.

- In a saucepan, brown the clove of garlic in a couple of tablespoons of extra-virgin olive oil. When we smell its scent in the kitchen, it is time to eliminate it and add the Tropea onion, sliced in icing, which we will make wither, paying attention to do not burn it, salting in moderation, on a very low flame.

- Add the banana and the diced chicken to the pot and mix the ingredients by "toasting": when the chicken starts to take on color, we raise the flame and add the white wine, cooking until it has completely evaporated. When the wine has evaporated, add the kale strips to the vegetables and chicken, mix gently and cook for a couple of minutes before serving with a generous sprinkle of pepper.

Nutrition:

- **Calories:** 525

Baked Salmon Fillet with Vegetable Garnish

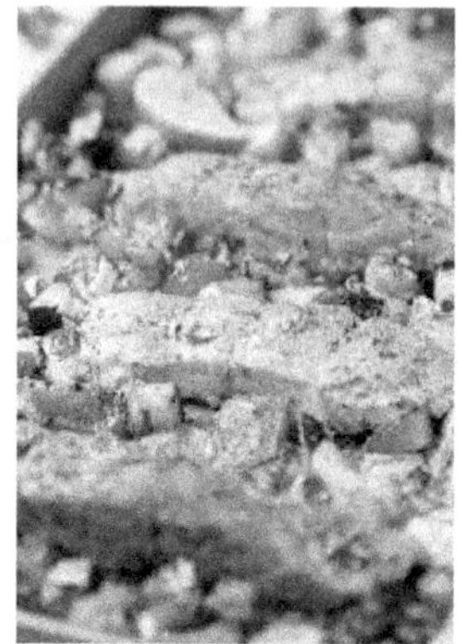

Preparation time: 20 minutes.

Cooking time: 30 minutes.

Servings: 4

Ingredients:

- 800 grams fillets of fresh salmon

- Dried oregano to taste

- 2 Big peppers

- 2 large green courgettes

- 3 large leeks

- 2 large carrots

- 2 tablespoons extra-virgin olive oil

- Salt to taste

- Chili pepper (optional)

Directions:

- To prepare this second fish dish with vegetables, we first prepare the vegetables that we can cook either in a pan, not fried, but steamed or baked.

- Finally, you just have to cook the 4 salmon fillets laying them on a baking tray, lined with parchment paper, sprinkling only with a little dry oregano (I don't add any oil or salt, I like that way).

- Bake in a preheated oven at 200°F for about 20/30 minutes, take out of the oven, remove the skin underneath the fillet (if present), lay each slice on the serving dish, and add the vegetable side dish before serving hot. Enjoy your meal!

Nutrition:

- **Calories:** 525

Buckwheat Spaghetti with Shrimp and Vegetables

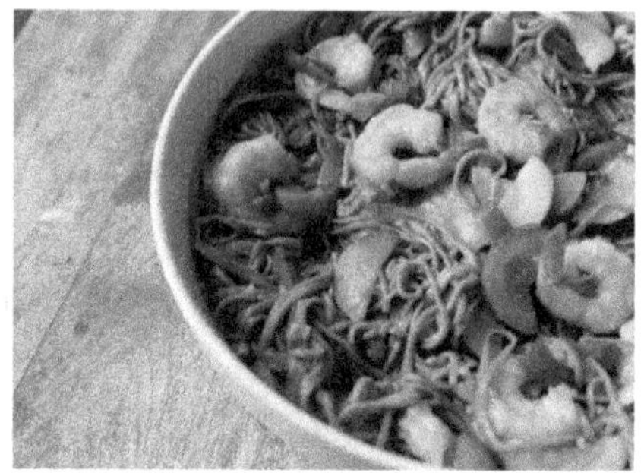

Preparation time: 15 minutes.

Cooking time: 20 minutes.

Servings: 4

Ingredients:

- 400 grams of Felicia buckwheat spaghetti

- 1 courgette

- 1 carrot

- 1 spring onion

- Ginger

- Extra-virgin olive oil to taste

- 1 carrot

- 100 grams of shrimp

- Salt to taste

- Soy sauce to taste

Directions:

- First, we grate the ginger, just 1 teaspoon, the spring onion and julienne the courgette and carrot and set everything aside. In a wok, put a tablespoon of olive oil, grated ginger and spring onion, and let it soften. Add the courgette and carrot in julienne strips and half a glass of water and leave to cook for just 5 minutes, they must be crunchy.

- Add the prawns and a generous spoonful of soy sauce and leave to cook for another 5 minutes and turn off and set aside. Meanwhile, cook the spaghetti in abundant salted water for the time indicated on the package, minus 1 minute. Drain and pour the spaghetti into the wok, add more soy sauce to taste and some spaghetti cooking water, and finish cooking in the wok.

- Serve in serving dishes and add more soy sauce to taste. Buckwheat noodles with shrimp and vegetables are ready.

Nutrition:

- **Calories:** 475

Risotto with Blueberries and Speck

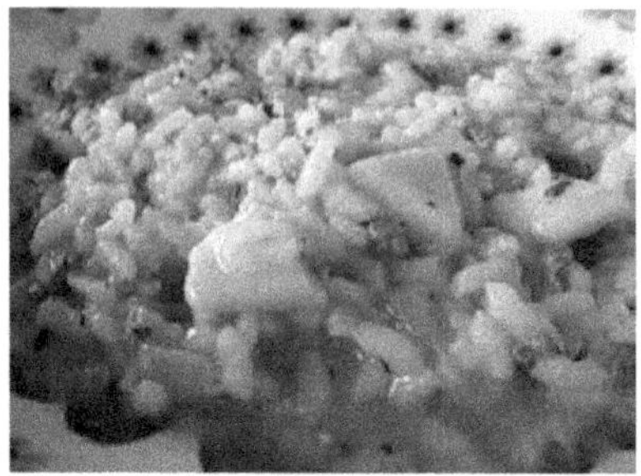

Preparation time: 15 minutes.

Cooking time: 25 minutes.

Servings: 2

Ingredients:

- 300 grams rice

- 200 grams blueberries

- 100 grams speck

- 1-liter vegetable broth

- 1 onion

- 4 tablespoons Grana Padano

- 40 grams butter

- Oil to taste

- Salt to taste

- Parsley to taste

Directions:

- Gently wash the blueberries and dry them with a towel.

- Cut the speck into strips without removing the fat part. Peel the onion and slice it finely with a knife.

- Heat the vegetable broth in a saucepan. Keep it on the heat over low heat so that it remains boiling but does not evaporate.

- Pour the oil into a pan, add the onion and let it dry on low heat. Add the rice and toast it for at least three minutes. Sprinkle with two ladles of hot broth. Stir and when the broth is absorbed, add a little more at a time.

- Cook for 10 minutes to add the blueberries and speck season with salt. Continue cooking for 10 minutes more. Wash the parsley and dry it thoroughly. Remove the leaves from the twigs, finely chop them with a knife or a crescent. Add the butter and parmesan and chopped parsley out of the heat. Let stand for two minutes with the lid on and serve accompanied with some parmesan wafers.

Nutrition:

- **Calories**: 530

Chapter 12: 7-Days Meal Plan

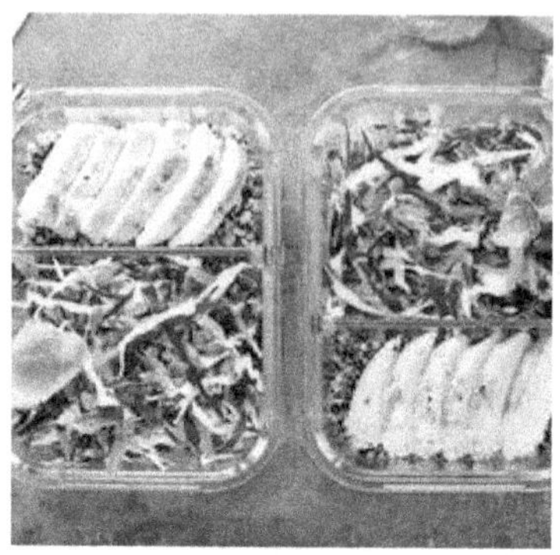

During this stage (the first three days of the meal plan), you need to have three green juices, so I suggest you have them at separate times of the day. To make it easier for you, have one drink in the morning, one in the midmorning, and one in the afternoon. If you remember, there is a rule stating that you need to drink the juice one or two hours after the meal. Well, during the first three days of the seven-day meal plan, you are entitled to only one main meal, and it is best to have it early during the day (the "eat early" principle). So, let's get into details:

Day 1

On this day, you can serve one main meal. You can choose either a vegan or a standard option. You can go for the miso and sesame-glazed tofu with chili stir-fried greens and ginger (vegan meal), or you can choose the standard option: buckwheat noodles with Asian shrimp stir-fry. You can have some dessert with these meals. You can have ½–¾ ounces of dark chocolate (85% cocoa). If you are having your meal at 7:00 a.m., then you can have the green juices at 8:30 a.m., 11:00 a.m., and 3:00 p.m.

Day 2

During this day, you will serve your juices at the same hours as the day before, and you can choose again for a vegan or standard meal. If the day before you had the standard meal, I would suggest the vegan meal on day 2, or if you had the vegan meal on day 1, then on this day, you can have the standard meal. However, this is up to you and your preferences, as nobody will blame you if you prefer just vegan or standard meals. So, here's what's on the menu for this day: turkey escalope with capers, parsley, sage, and spiced cauliflower "couscous" (standard) or kale with buckwheat and red onion dal (vegan).

You can serve the same dessert as the previous day, respecting the recommended quantity.

Day 3

You can continue the same schedule when it comes to your meal and green juices. You can even choose the same dessert. However, there is something different in the menu for the day: cauliflower "couscous" with harissa baked tofu (vegan) or aromatic chicken breast with red onions, kale, and chili and tomato salsa.

This part of the first week is less radical than the previous one, but it involves lowering your green juice intake from three servings to just two. You can have one green juice at 9:00 a.m. and the second one at 4:00 p.m. (for instance), but you can adjust the schedule according to your time. But don't worry. As you will compensate with an extra main meal, you will have two meals per day during this phase. You should be able to keep the same dessert (the dark chocolate with 85 percent cocoa), and you will have again the option to choose from a standard or vegan meal.

Day 4

For this day, you will have included in your menu two standard meals and two vegan meals. You can choose to have both meals standard and both meals vegan, but if you want to mix them (to have one meal vegan and the other one standard), feel free to do so. You can have your breakfast at 7:00 a.m. and the second meal at 1:00 p.m.

Therefore, these are the regular meals: sirt muesli, which is a proper breakfast meal, and salmon fillet with caramelized endive, celery leaf, and arugula salad. (Don't forget to pour some extra-virgin olive oil on the salad).

As for the vegan meals, you can have sirt muesli (vegan style) and Tuscan bean stew.

Day 5

For this day, you can stick to the same juice drinking and eating schedule. The only difference is that you are trying different meals than the day before.

For the standard diet, you can have strawberry buckwheat tabbouleh and stir-fried greens with miso-marinated baked cod. For the vegan menu, you can try vegan strawberry buckwheat tabbouleh and buckwheat noodles in miso broth with celery, kale, and tofu.

Day 6

There isn't too much difference between day 6 and the previous days of phase 2. Just stick to the same green juices and the same schedule for having them, or you can have the meals.

When it comes to the standard food preference, you can have sirt super salad and grilled beef with herb-roasted potatoes, onion rings, garlic kale, and red wine. (Now this sounds too delicious, so you have to try it).

But if you are not into beef, then perhaps you want to go with the vegan menu: lentil sirt super salad and baked potato with kidney bean mole.

Day 7

You are finishing the seven-day meal plan in style, as this day has included incredibly delicious meals. You already have the scheduled set for your meals and green juices, plus you still have a small piece of dark chocolate (after each meal) to sweeten your day (not that it requires sweetening).

If you want to choose the regular meals, you can go with the sirtfood omelet, baked chicken breast with walnut, and red onion and parsley pesto salad (some extra-virgin olive oil is recommended). If you feel like you want to try the vegan menu, you can have vegan Waldorf salad and roasted eggplant wedges with walnut and tomato and parsley pesto salad (don't forget to add extra-virgin olive oil).

The menu suggested during these days can be used as guidelines. Still, it is up to you if you want to stick to having these meals precisely on the same days as mentioned in the plan. Perhaps you want to try the meal from day 1 to day 3, and the other way around. I wouldn't recommend trying a meal from day 5 or day 6 in phase 1 of the seven-day meal plan. Therefore, feel free to play with the meals, but make sure you don't have a phase 2 meal from week in phase 1 or the other way around. You will need to pay attention to quantity as well. These foods may sound delicious, but you can't have a considerable portion. You need to stick with the quantity mentioned in the recipes.

Chapter 13: Desserts Recipes

Fruit Skewers & Strawberry Dip

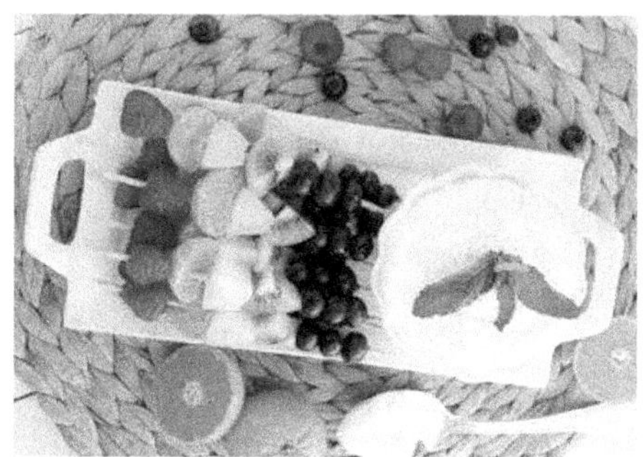

Preparation time: 15 minutes.

Cooking time: 0 minutes.

Servings: 4

Ingredients:

- 150 grams (5 ounces) red grapes

- 1 pineapple, (approx. 2 pounds weight) peeled and diced

- 400 grams (14 ounces) strawberries

Directions:

- Place 100 grams (3(½) ounces) of the strawberries into a food processor and blend until smooth. Pour the dip into a serving bowl. Skewer the grapes, pineapple chunks and the remaining strawberries onto skewers. Serve alongside the strawberry dip.

Nutrition:

- **Calories:** 147

Choc Nut Truffles

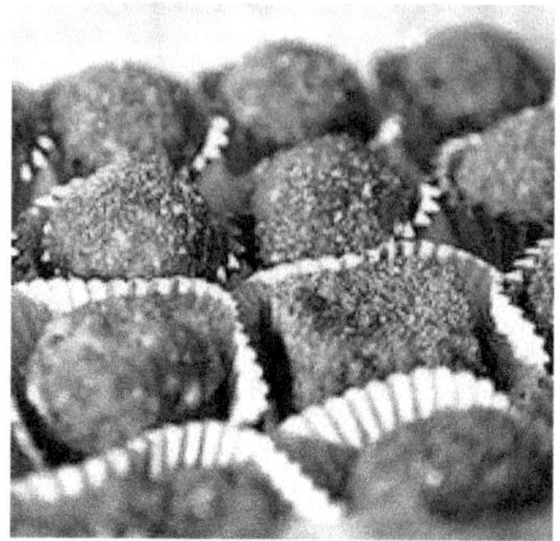

Preparation time: 15 minutes.

Cooking time: 0 minutes.

Servings: 8

Ingredients:

- 150 grams (5 ounces) desiccated (shredded) coconut

- 50 grams (2 ounces) walnuts, chopped

- 25 grams (1 ounce) hazelnuts, chopped

- 4 Medjool dates

- 2 tablespoons 100% cocoa powder or cacao nibs

- 1 tablespoon coconut oil

Directions:

- Place all the ingredients into a blender and process until smooth and creamy. Using a teaspoon, scoop the mixture into bite-size pieces, then roll it into balls. Place them into small paper cases, cover them and chill for 1 hour before serving.

Nutrition:

- **Calories:** 236

No-Bake Strawberry Flapjacks

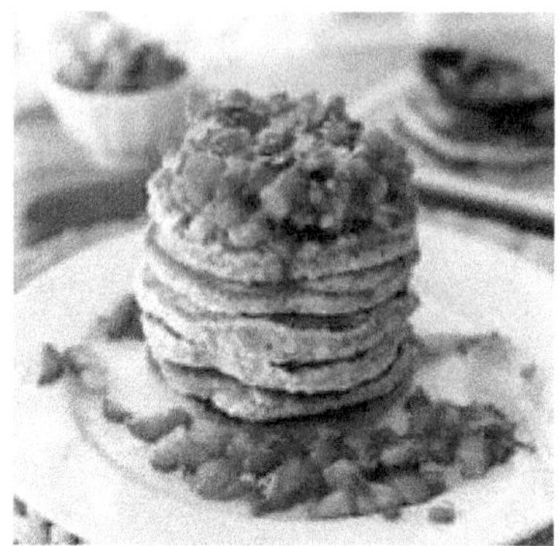

Preparation time: 15 minutes.

Cooking time: 0 minutes.

Servings: 8

Ingredients

- 75 grams (3 ounces) porridge oats

- 125 grams (4 ounces) dates

- 50 grams (2 ounces) strawberries

- 50 grams (2 ounces) peanuts (unsalted)

- 50 grams (2 ounces) walnuts

- 1 tablespoon coconut oil

- 2 tablespoons 100% cocoa powder or cacao nibs

Directions:

- Place all the ingredients into a blender and process until they become a soft consistency. Spread the mixture onto a baking sheet or small flat tin. Press the mixture down and smooth it out. Cut it into 8 pieces, ready to serve. You can add an extra sprinkling of cocoa powder to garnish if you wish.

Nutrition:

- **Calories:** 182

Chocolate Balls

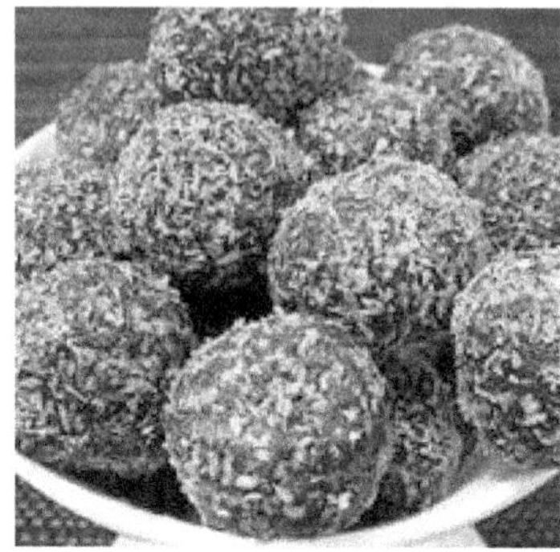

Preparation time: 15 minutes.

Cooking time: 0 minutes.

Servings: 6

Ingredients:

- 50 grams (2 ounces) peanut butter (or almond butter)

- 25 grams (1 ounce) cocoa powder

- 25 grams (1 ounce) desiccated (shredded) coconut

- 1 tablespoon honey

- 1 tablespoon cocoa powder for coating

Direction:

- Place the ingredients into a bowl and mix. Using a teaspoon, scoop out a little of the mixture and shape it into a ball. Roll the ball in a little cocoa powder and set it aside. Repeat for the remaining mixture. They can be eaten straight away or stored in the fridge.

Nutrition:

- **Calories:** 115

Warm Berries & Cream

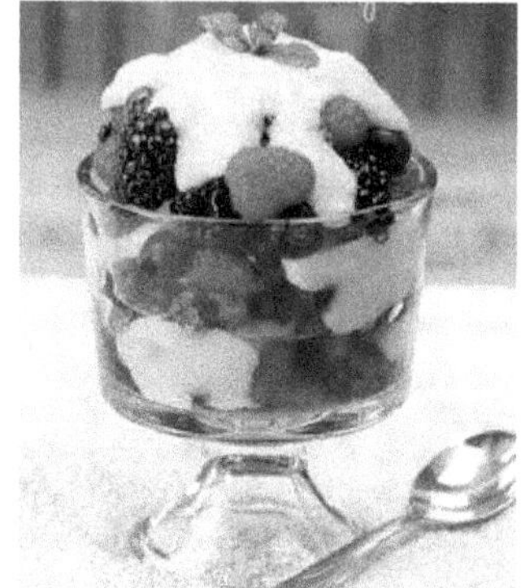

Preparation time: 15 minutes.

Cooking time: 0 minutes.

Servings: 4

Ingredients:

- 250 grams (9 ounces) blueberries

- 250 grams (9 ounces) strawberries

- 100 grams (3(½) ounces) redcurrants

- 100 grams (3(½) ounces) blackberries

- 4 tablespoons fresh whipped cream

- 1 tablespoon honey

- Zest and juice of 1 orange

Directions:

- Place all the berries into a pan along with the honey and orange juice. Gently heat the berries for around 5 minutes until warmed through. Serve the berries into bowls and add a dollop of whipped cream on top. Alternatively, you could top them off with fromage frais or yogurt.

Nutrition:

- **Calories:** 180

Chocolate Fondue

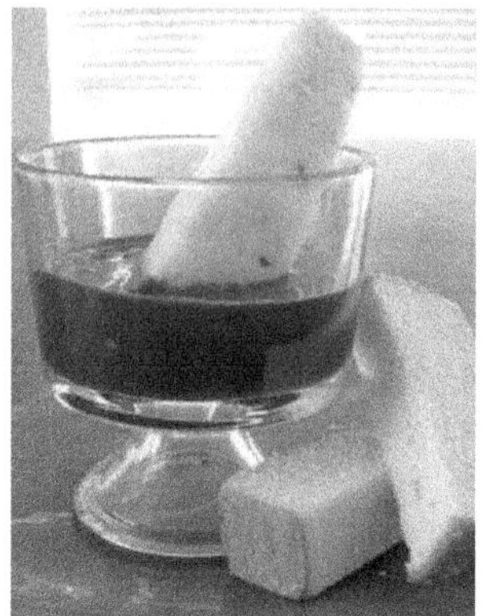

Preparation time: 5 minutes.

Cooking time: 0 minutes.

Servings: 4

Ingredients:

- 125 grams (4 ounces) dark chocolate (minimum 85% cocoa)

- 300 grams (11 ounces) strawberries

- 200 grams (7 ounces) cherries

- 2 apples, peeled, cored and sliced

- 100 milliliters (3(½) ounces) double cream (heavy cream)

Directions:

- Place the chocolate and cream into a fondue pot or saucepan and warm it until smooth and creamy. Serve in the fondue pot or transfer it to a serving bowl. Scatter the fruit on a serving dish ready to be dipped into the chocolate.

Nutrition:

- **Calories:** 352

Walnut & Date Loaf

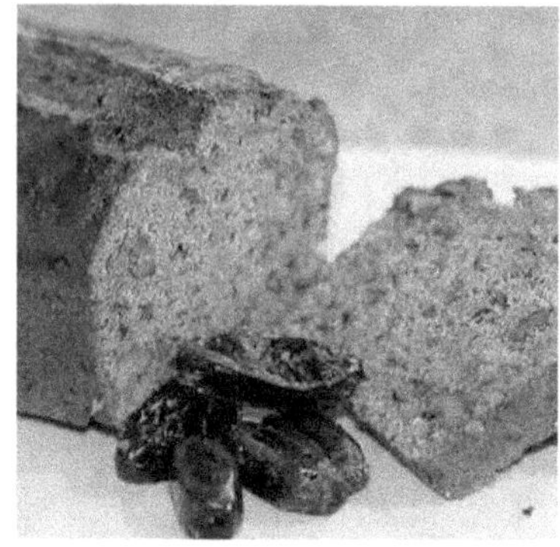

Preparation time: 10 minutes.

Cooking time: 45 minutes.

Servings: 12

Ingredients:

- 250 grams (9 ounces) self-rising flour

- 125 grams (4 ounces) Medjool dates, chopped

- 50 grams (2 ounces) walnuts, chopped

- 250 milliliters (8fl ounces) milk

- 3 eggs

- 1 medium banana, mashed

- 1 teaspoon baking soda

Directions:

- Sieve the baking soda and flour into a bowl. Add in the banana, eggs, milk and dates and combine all the ingredients thoroughly. Transfer the mixture to a lined loaf tin and smooth it out. Scatter the walnuts on top. Bake the loaf in the oven at 180°C/360°F for 45 minutes. Transfer it to a wire rack to cool before serving.

Nutrition:

- **Calories:** 166

Strawberry Frozen Yogurt

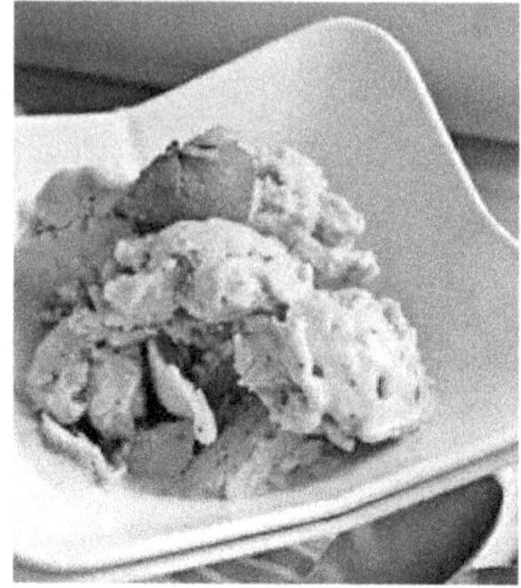

Preparation time: 3 hours.

Cooking time: 0 minutes.

Servings: 4

Ingredients:

- 450 grams (1 pound) plain yogurt

- 175 grams (6 ounces) strawberries

- Juice of 1 orange

- 1 tablespoon honey

Directions:

- Place the strawberries and orange juice into a food processor or blender and blitz until smooth. Press the mixture through a sieve into a large bowl to remove seeds. Stir in the honey and yogurt. Transfer the mixture to an ice-cream maker and follow the machine's instructions. Alternatively, pour the mixture into a container and place it in the fridge for 1 hour. Use a fork to whisk it and break up ice crystals and freeze for 2 hours.

Nutrition:

- **Calories:** 133

Chocolate Brownies

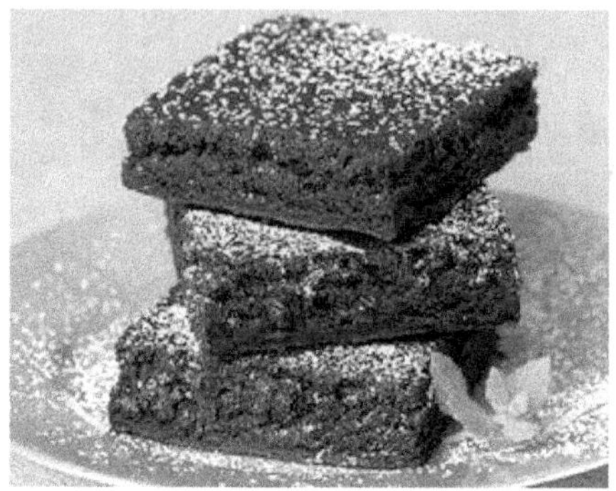

Preparation time: 15 minutes.

Cooking time: 25–30 minutes.

Servings: 14

Ingredients:

- 200 grams (7 ounces) dark chocolate (minimum 85% cocoa)

- 200 grams (7 ounces) Medjool dates, stone removed

- 100 grams (3(½) ounces) walnuts, chopped

- 3 eggs

- 25 milliliters (1 fl ounces) melted coconut oil

- 2 teaspoons vanilla essence

- ½ teaspoon baking soda

Directions:

- Place the dates, chocolate, eggs, coconut oil, baking soda and vanilla essence into a food processor and mix until smooth. Stir the walnuts into the mixture. Pour the mixture into a shallow baking tray. Transfer to the oven and bake at 180°C/350°F for 25–30 minutes. Allow it to cool. Cut into pieces and serve.

Nutrition:

- **Calories:** 197

Crème Brûlée

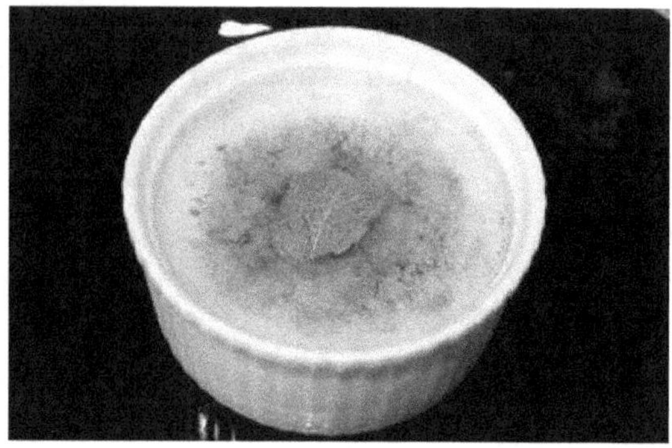

Preparation time: 15 minutes.

Cooking time: 3–5 minutes.

Servings: 4

Ingredients

- 400 grams (14 ounces) strawberries

- 300 grams (11 ounces) plain low-fat yogurt

- 125 grams (4 ounces) Greek yogurt

- 100 grams (3(½) ounces) brown sugar

- 1 teaspoon vanilla extract

Directions:

- Divide the strawberries between 4 ramekin dishes. In a bowl, combine the plain yogurt with the vanilla extract. Spoon the mixture onto the strawberries. Scoop the Greek yogurt on top. Sprinkle the sugar into each ramekin dish, completely covering the top. Place the dishes under a hot grill (broiler) for around 3 minutes or until the sugar has caramelized.

Nutrition:

- **Calories:** 213

Pistachio Fudge

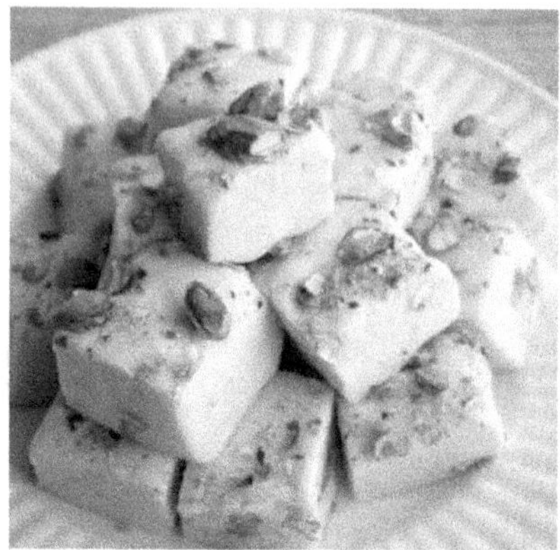

Preparation time: 15 minutes.

Cooking time: 0 minutes.

Servings: 10

Ingredients

- 225 grams (8 ounces) Medjool dates

- 100 grams (3(½) ounces) pistachio nuts, shelled (or other nuts)

- 50 grams (2 ounces) desiccated (shredded) coconut

- 25 grams (1 ounce) oats

- 2 tablespoons water

Directions:

- Place the dates, nuts, coconut, oats and water into a food processor and process until the ingredients are well mixed.

Remove the mixture and roll it to 2 centimeters (1 inch) thick. Cut it into 10 pieces and serve.

Nutrition:

- **Calories:** 162

Spiced Poached Apples

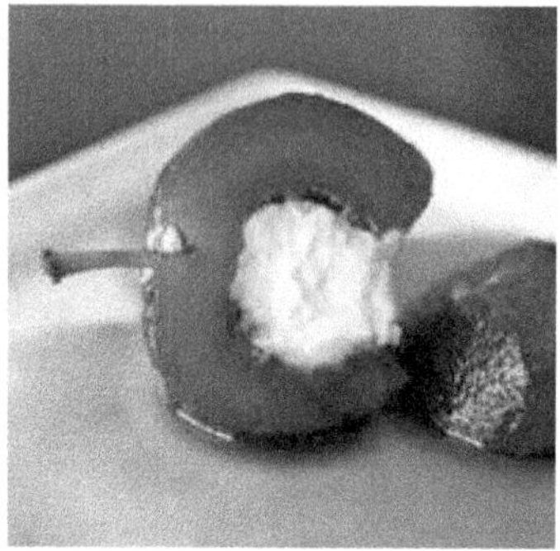

Preparation time: 15 minutes.

Cooking time: 15 minutes.

Servings: 4

Ingredients

- 4 apples

- 2 tablespoons honey

- 4-star anise

- 2 cinnamon sticks

- 300 milliliters (½ pint) green tea

Directions:

- Place the honey and green tea into a saucepan and bring to the boil. Add the apples, star anise and cinnamon. Reduce the heat and simmer gently for 15 minutes. Serve the apples with a dollop of crème fraiche or Greek yogurt.

Nutrition:

- **Calories**: 99

Chapter 14: Bonus Recipe

Sirtfood Cauliflower Couscous & Turkey Steak

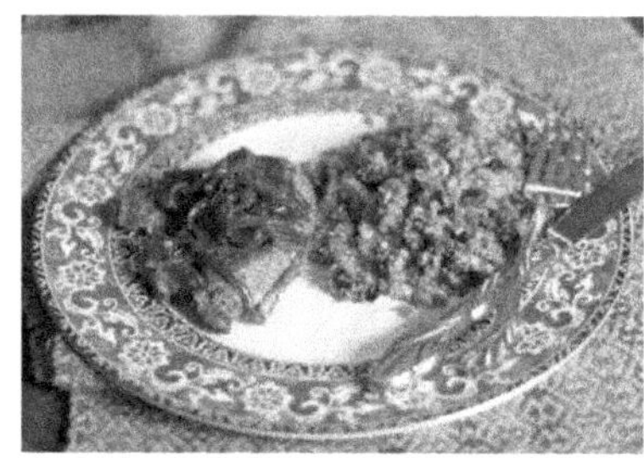

Preparation time: 15 minutes.

Cooking time: 10 minutes.

Servings: 6

Ingredients:

- 150 grams cauliflower, roughly chopped

- 1 garlic clove, finely chopped

- 40 grams red onion, finely chopped

- 1 bird's-eye chili, finely chopped

- 1 teaspoon finely chopped fresh ginger

- 2 tablespoons extra-virgin olive oil

- 2 teaspoons ground turmeric

- 30 grams sun-dried tomatoes, finely chopped

- 10 grams parsley

- 150 grams turkey steak

- 1 teaspoon dried sage

- Juice of ½ lemon

- 1 tablespoon capers

Directions:

- Blend in 1–2 pulses until the cauliflower has a breadcrumb-like consistency.

- In a skillet, fry garlic, chili, ginger and red onion in 1 teaspoon olive oil for 2–3 minutes. Throw in the turmeric and cauliflower, then cook for another 1–2 minutes. Remove from heat and add the tomatoes and roughly half the parsley.

- Garnish the turkey steak with sage and dress with oil. In a skillet, over medium heat, fry the turkey steak for 5 minutes, turning occasionally. Once the steak is cooked, add lemon juice, capers and a dash of water. Stir and serve with the couscous.

Nutrition:

- **Calories:** 112

Sirtfood Granola

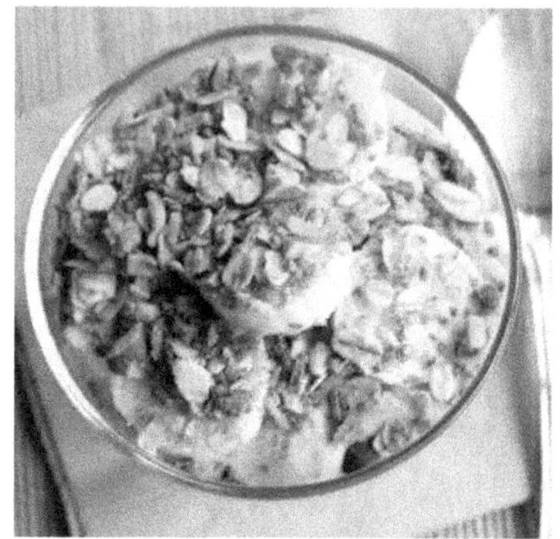

Preparation time: 25 minutes.

Cooking time: 50 minutes.

Servings: 6

Ingredients:

- 200 grams oats

- 250 grams buckwheat flakes

- 100 grams walnuts, chopped

- 100 grams almonds, chopped

- 100 grams dried strawberries

- 1(½) teaspoon ground ginger

- 1(½) teaspoon ground cinnamon

- 120 milliliters olive oil

- 2 tablespoons honey

Directions:

- Preheat oven to 150°C or gas mark 3. Line a tray with baking parchment.

- Stir together walnuts, almonds, buckwheat flakes and oats with ginger and cinnamon. In a large pan, warm olive oil and honey, heating until the honey has dissolved.

- Pour the honey-oil over the other ingredients. Separate the granola evenly over the lined baking tray and roast for 50 minutes, or until golden.

- Remove from the oven and leave to cool. Once cooled, add the berries and store them in an airtight container. Eat dry or with milk and yogurt. It stays fresh for up to 1 week.

Nutrition:

- **Calories:** 536

Red Onion Dhal

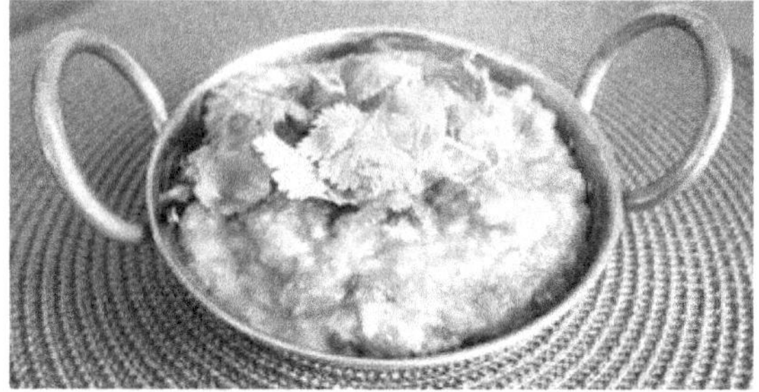

Preparation time: 25 minutes.

Cooking time: 30 minutes.

Servings: 4

Ingredients:

- 1 teaspoon extra-virgin olive oil

- 1 teaspoon mustard seeds

- 40 grams red onion, finely chopped

- 1 garlic clove, finely chopped

- 1 teaspoon finely chopped fresh ginger

- 1 bird's-eye chili, finely chopped

- 1 teaspoon mild curry powder

- 2 teaspoons ground turmeric

- 300 milliliters vegetable stock

- 40 grams red lentils, rinsed

- 50 grams kale

- 50 milliliters tinned coconut milk

- 50 grams buckwheat

Directions:

- In a moderately sized saucepan, warm the olive oil over medium heat. Toss in the mustard seeds and fry until they start to crackle. Add the garlic, ginger, chili and onion frying for 10 minutes, or until the onion is tender.

- Throw in 1 teaspoon turmeric and curry powder and then stir. Cook for a few minutes until fragrant, then pour in the stock and bring to the boil. Pour in the lentils and cook for 30 minutes.

- Add the coconut milk and kale, cooking for another 5 minutes or so. As the dhal is brewing, rinse the buckwheat with water and cook it according to packet instructions. Drain and serve with the dhal.

Nutrition:

- **Calories:** 27

Miso Caramelized Tofu

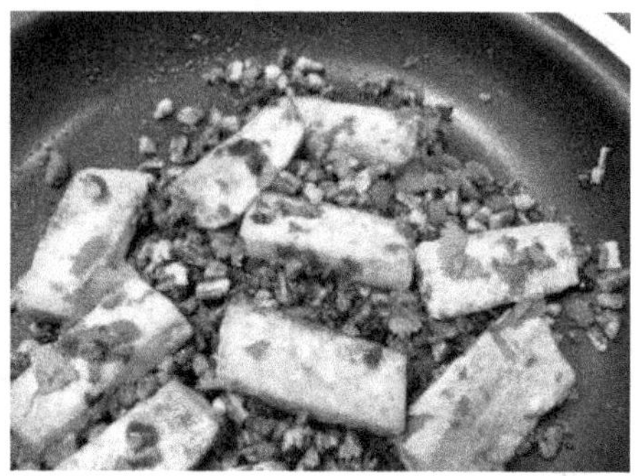

Preparation time: 15 minutes.

Cooking time: 25 minutes.

Servings: 6

Ingredients:

- 1 tablespoon mirin

- 20 grams miso paste

- 1*150 grams firm tofu

- 40 grams celery, trimmed

- 35 grams red onion

- 120 grams courgette

- 1 bird's-eye chili

- 1 garlic clove, finely chopped

- 1 teaspoon finely chopped fresh ginger

- 50 grams kale, chopped

- 2 teaspoons sesame seeds

- 35 grams buckwheat

- 1 teaspoon ground turmeric

- 2 teaspoons extra-virgin olive oil

- 1 teaspoon tamari (or soy sauce)

Directions:

- Pre-heat your over to 200°C or gas mark 6. Cover a tray with baking parchment.

- Combine the mirin and miso. Dice the tofu and coat it in the mirin-miso mixture in a reusable plastic bag. Set aside to marinate.

- Chop the vegetables (except for the kale) at a diagonal angle to produce long slices. Using a steamer, cook for the kale for 5 minutes and set aside.

- Disperse the tofu across the lined tray and garnish with sesame seeds. Roast for 20 minutes or until caramelized.

- Rinse the buckwheat using running water and a sieve. Add to a pan of boiling water alongside turmeric and cook the buckwheat according to the packet instructions.

- Heat the oil in a skillet over high heat. Toss in the vegetables, herbs and spices, then fry for 2–3 minutes. Reduce to medium heat and fry for a further 5 minutes or until cooked but still crunchy.

Nutrition:

- **Calories:** 198

Prawn & Chili Pak Choi

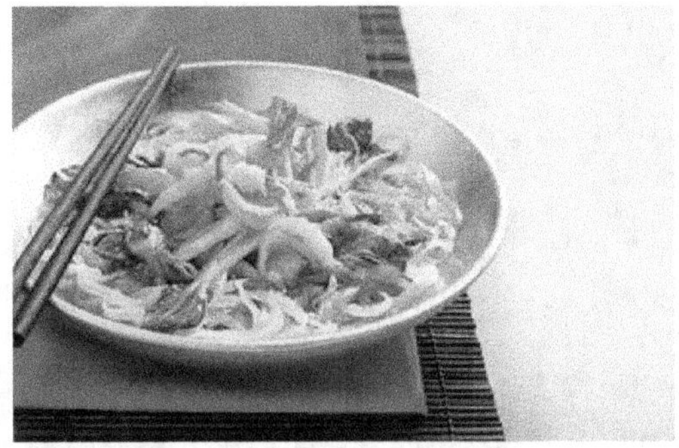

Preparation time: 35 minutes.

Cooking time: 30–45 minutes.

Servings: 4

Ingredients:

- 75 grams brown rice

- 1 pak choi

- 60 milliliters chicken stock

- 1 tablespoon extra-virgin olive oil

- 1 garlic clove, finely chopped

- 50 grams red onion, finely chopped

- ½ bird's-eye chili, finely chopped

- 1 teaspoon freshly grated ginger

- 125 grams shelled raw king prawns

- 1 tablespoon soy sauce

- 1 teaspoon five-spice

- 1 tablespoon freshly chopped flat-leaf parsley

- A pinch of salt and pepper

Directions:

- Bring a medium-sized saucepan of water to the boil and cook the brown rice for 25–30 minutes, or until softened.

- Tear the pak choi into pieces. Warm the chicken stock in a skillet over medium heat and toss in the pak choi, cooking until the pak choi has slightly wilted.

- In another skillet, warm olive oil over high heat. Toss in the ginger, chili, red onions, and garlic frying for 2–3 minutes.

- Throw in the pawns, five-spice and soy sauce and cook for 6–8 minutes, or until cooked throughout. Drain the brown rice and add to the skillet, stirring and cooking for 2–3 minutes. Add the pak choi, garnish with parsley and serve.

Nutrition:

- **Calories:** 12

King Prawn Stir-Fry & Soba

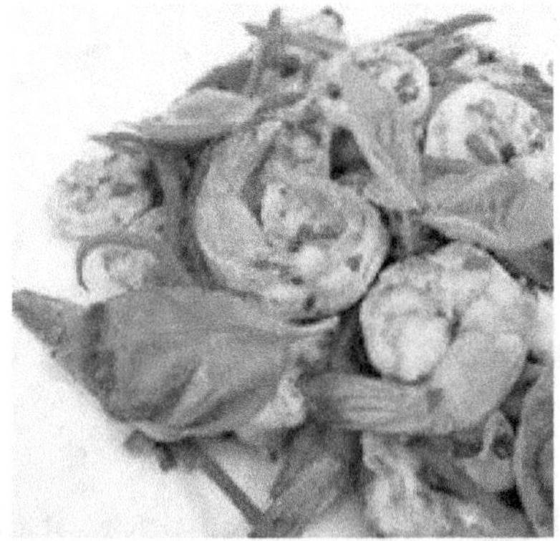

Preparation time: 15 minutes.

Cooking time: 5 minutes.

Servings: 6

Ingredients:

- 150 grams shelled raw king prawns, deveined

- 2 teaspoons tamaris

- 2 teaspoons extra-virgin olive oil

- 75 grams soba

- 1 garlic clove, finely chopped

- 1 bird's-eye chili, finely chopped

- 1 teaspoon finely chopped fresh ginger

- 20 grams red onions, sliced

- 40 grams celery, trimmed and sliced

- 75 grams green beans, chopped

- 50 grams kale, roughly chopped

- 100 milliliters chicken stock

Directions:

- Warm a skillet over high heat and then fry the pawns in 1 teaspoon of the tamari and 1 teaspoon of olive oil. Transfer the contents of the skillet to a plate and then wipe the skillet with the kitchen towel to remove the lingering sauce.

- Boil water and cook the soba for 8 minutes or according to packet instructions. Drain and set aside for future use. Using the remaining 1 teaspoon olive oil, fry the remaining ingredients for 3–4 minutes. Add the stock and bring to the boil, simmering until the vegetables are tender but still have a bite.

- Add the lavage, noodles and prawn into the skillet, stir, bring back to the boil and then serve.

Nutrition:

- **Calories**: 99

Tomato Frittata

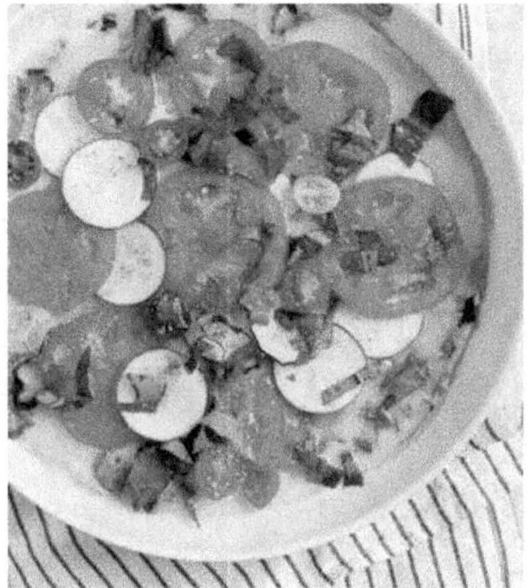

Preparation time: 15 minutes.

Cooking time: 10-15 minutes.

Servings: 4

Ingredients:

- 50 grams cheddar cheese, grated

- 75 grams Kalamata olives, pitted and halved

- 8 cherry tomatoes, halved

- 4 large eggs

- 1 tablespoon fresh parsley, chopped

- 1 tablespoon fresh basil, chopped

- 1 tablespoon olive oil

Directions:

Whisk eggs together in a large mixing bowl. Toss in the parsley, basil, olives, tomatoes and cheese, stirring thoroughly.

In a small skillet, heat the olive oil over high heat. Pour in the frittata mixture and cook for 5–10 minutes or set. Remove the skillet from the hob and place under the grill for 5 minutes, or until firm and set. Divide into portions and serve immediately.

Nutrition:

- **Calories** 79

Tofu & Shiitake Mushroom Soup

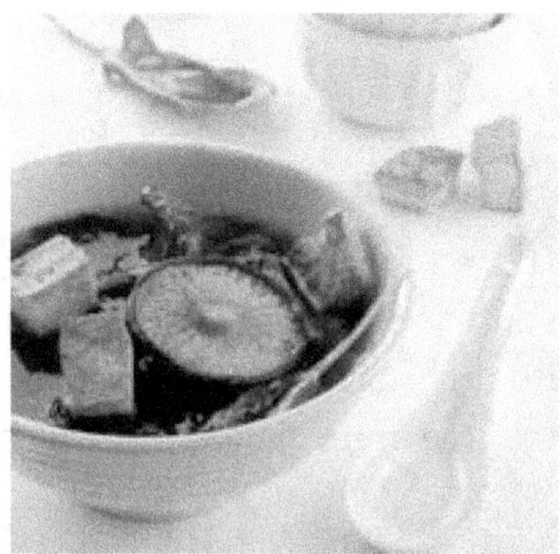

Preparation time: 15 minutes.

Cooking time: 10 minutes.

Servings: 6

Ingredients

- 10 grams dried wakame

- 1-liter vegetable stock

- 200 grams shiitake mushrooms, sliced

- 120 grams miso paste

- 1*400 grams firm tofu, diced

- 2 green onions, trimmed and diagonally chopped

- 1 bird's-eye chili, finely chopped

Directions:

- Soak the wakame in lukewarm water for 10–15 minutes before draining.

- In a medium-sized saucepan, add the vegetable stock and bring to the boil. Toss in the mushrooms and simmer for 2–3 minutes.

- Mix the miso paste with 3–4 tablespoon of vegetable stock from the saucepan until the miso is entirely dissolved. Pour the miso-stock back into the pan and add the tofu, wakame, green onions and chili, then serve immediately.

Nutrition:

- **Calories:** 98

Horseradish Flaked Salmon Fillet & Kale

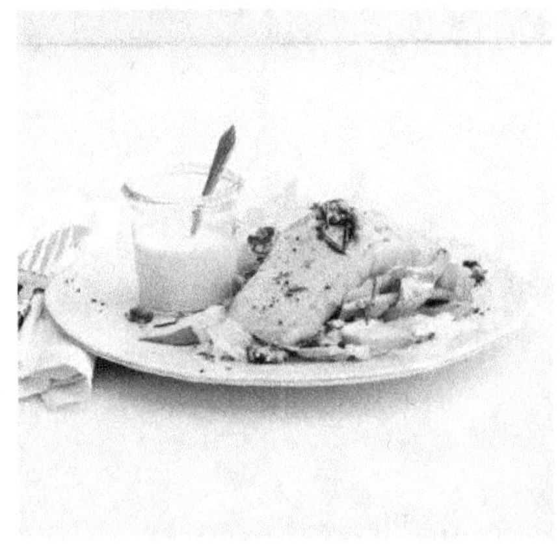

Preparation time: 25 minutes.

Cooking time: 10–15 minutes.

Servings: 6

Ingredients:

- 200 grams skinless, boneless salmon fillet

- 50 grams green beans

- 75 grams kale

- 1 tablespoon extra-virgin olive oil

- ½ garlic clove, crushed

- 50 grams red onion, chopped

- 1 tablespoon fresh chives, chopped

- 1 tablespoon freshly chopped flat-leaf parsley

- 1 tablespoon low fat crème fraiche

- 1 tablespoon horseradish sauce

- Juice of ¼ lemon

- A pinch of salt and pepper

Directions:

- Preheat the grill.

- Sprinkle a salmon fillet with salt and pepper. Place under the grill for 10–15 minutes. Flake and set aside.

- Using a steamer, cook the kale and green beans for 10 minutes.

- In a skillet, warm the oil over high heat. Add garlic and red onion and fry for 23 minutes. Toss in the kale and beans and then cook for 1–2 minutes more.

- Mix the chives, parsley, crème fraiche, horseradish, lemon juice and flaked salmon.

- Serve the kale and beans topped with the dressed flaked salmon.

Nutrition:

- **Calories:** 902

Mushroom & Tofu Scramble

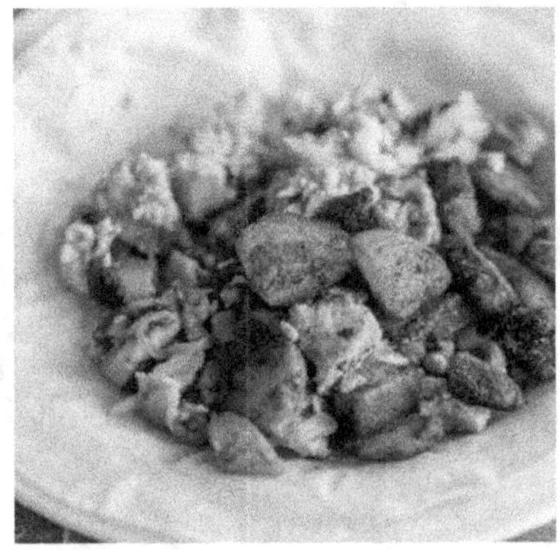

Preparation time: 15 minutes.

Cooking time: 10 minutes.

Servings: 8

Ingredients:

- 100 grams tofu, extra firm

- 1 teaspoon ground turmeric

- 1 teaspoon mild curry powder

- 20 grams kale, roughly chopped

- 1 teaspoon extra-virgin olive oil

- 20 grams red onion, thinly sliced

- 50 grams mushrooms, thinly sliced

- 5 grams parsley, finely chopped

- Chili

Directions:

- Place 2 sheets of kitchen towel under and on top of the tofu, then rest a considerable weight such as saucepan onto the tofu, to ensure it drains off the liquid.

- Combine the curry powder, turmeric and 1-2 teaspoon of water to form a paste. Using a steamer cook kale for 3–4 minutes.

- In a skillet, warm oil over medium heat. Add the chili, mushrooms and onion, cooking for several minutes or until brown and tender.

- Break the tofu into small pieces and toss in the skillet. Coat with the spice paste and stir, ensuring everything becomes evenly coated. Cook for up to 5 minutes, or until the tofu has browned, then add the kale and fry for 2 more minutes. Garnish with parsley before serving.

Nutrition:

- **Calories:** 105

Tuna Salad

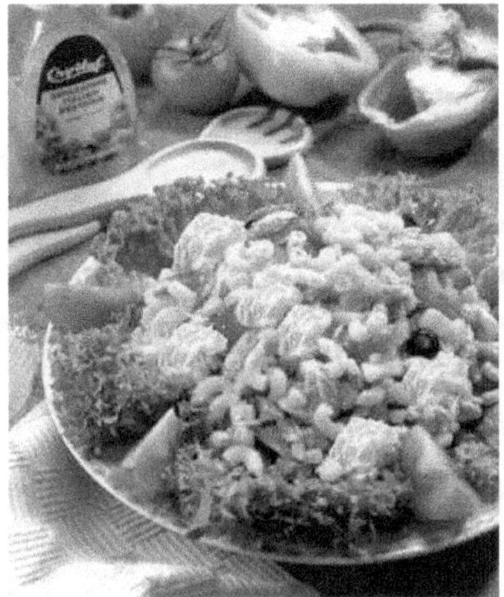

Preparation time: 5 minutes.

Cooking time: 0 minutes.

Servings: 8

Ingredients:

- 100 grams red chicory

- 150 grams tuna flakes in brine, drained

- 100 grams cucumber

- 25 grams rocket

- 6 Kalamata olives, pitted

- 2 hard-boiled eggs, peeled and quartered

- 2 tomatoes, chopped

- 2 tablespoons fresh parsley, chopped

- 1 red onion, chopped

- 1 celery stalk

- 1 tablespoon capers

- 2 tablespoons garlic vinaigrette

Directions:

- Combine all the ingredients in a bowl and serve.

Nutrition:

- **Calories:** 100

Conclusion

Before ending this book, most of you are probably curious about the safety and potential side effects of the Sirt diet, as you should be. To put it simply, the safety and whether you experience side effects all depend on your health and what day-to-day choices you may, just like it does on any diet. The Sirt diet is usually safe. However, there are some cautions you should keep in mind to have the best experience possible.

Foods rich in sirtuins are also incredibly helpful superfoods that anyone could benefit from eating more of. They are high in anti-inflammatory properties and antioxidants, both of which can reduce the risk of disease and slow down cellular aging. But, if you only choose to eat foods on the Sirt food list I have provided you above, then you will not be eating a balanced diet. This is why the recipes in this book also include other fruits, vegetables, grains, and protein sources. You cannot live off of only a handful of ingredients, at least not healthfully. If you try to eat only sirtuin-rich foods, you may lose more health in the short-term, but you will only experience adverse long-term side effects. This is why I, again and again, promote the importance of eating a balanced Sirtfood diet.

The first phase of the Sirt diet can be restrictive, as you are eating one thousand to fifteen hundred calories a day. However, for this reason, the first phase only lasts a week and is healthy to do in the short-term. You wouldn't want to live an entire month eating that number of calories a day, but for a week most, it is sufficient for most people. Regularly consult your family doctor before making significant life changes that affect your health. Depending on your specific health, weight, and activity level, you might need to adjust a diet plan to make it work for your individual needs.

Your doctor is the one most qualified to determine if you need to make these given adjustments. For instance, if you work a manual labor job, your doctor might recommend you increase your calorie and protein intake to keep your energy levels up. Remember, if your doctor does have concerns due to your health, it doesn't mean you can't follow the Sirt diet, simply that you need to make their recommended adjustments to your plan.

Thankfully, the average healthy adult is unlikely to have any problems with the Sirt diet if they follow it in a balanced manner recommended. This means you shouldn't increase the duration of phase one to promote further weight loss. Remember, if you want to lose more weight, then only repeat phase one after completing phase two. For a healthy adult, the most common side effects are fatigue, irritability, and lightheadedness. This is usually due to calorie restriction and can occur whenever a person goes on a diet or changes their eating habits. You should also know that this diet is not recommended for anyone with an eating disorder.

This is because while the calorie restriction is healthy when followed according to plan, for a person who already has disordered eating, it only reinforces their negative relationship with food. The result could be that if someone with an eating disorder attempts to follow this or any other diet calling for counting calories that their eating disorder will likely worsen. Of course, if you or someone you know has an eating disorder and still wants to benefit from Sirtuin-rich foods, you can still enjoy the recipes in this book and incorporate the top Sirtfoods into your daily meal plan without cutting your calorie intake. You may not experience as much weight loss. Still, you have to prioritize your mental health and healing from disordered eating.

To sum it up, you should speak with your doctor before drastically changing your eating habits no matter what diet you are trying, including the Sirt diet. However, if you are healthy and not pregnant, breastfeeding, or suffering from an eating disorder, it should be safe if you follow the diet as recommended. Even if you have a chronic illness or disease, it may be healthy. Still, only your doctor can say for sure, as each person's disease, condition, and treatment will vary.